Day Six

When Motherhood and Madness Collide

First published in 2013 by Green Olive Press
PO Box 1417
Woollahra NSW 1350
www.greenolivepress.com

Copyright © Jen S. Wight 2013

Jen S. Wight asserts the moral right to be identified as the author of this book.
All rights reserved. No part of this book may be reproduced or transmitted in any form or by any means, electronic or mechanical, including photocopying, recording or by any other information storage or retrieval system, without prior permission in writing from the publisher.

National Library of Australia
Cataloguing-in-Publication entry

    Author: Wight, Jen, author.
    Title: Day six : when motherhood and madness collide / Jen Wight ;
    Illustrator: Bhavna Khanna.
    ISBN: 9780987209979 (paperback)
        Postpartum depression--Patients--Biography.
        Postpartum depression--Patients--Family relationships.
        Postpartum depression--Treatment.
        Postpartum psychiatric disorders.
        Depression in women--Patients--Biography.
        Mothers--Mental health.
    Other Authors/Contributors: Khanna, Bhavna, illustrator.
    Dewey Number: 618.76092

Cover and internal design: Gloria Tsang/Green Olive Press
Internal printing: McPhersons Printing Group

Day Six

When Motherhood & Madness Collide

For my little big sister

Praise for Day Six

This gripping book will take readers into the darkest of postpartum mood disorders. Despite the gravity of the topic and the torture that Jen describes over an extended period, she recounts her excruciating physical and mental experiences with irony, whimsy and sharp observations. Importantly, hers is a message of hope, and she itemises the key ingredients involved in coming out of the darkness of a postnatal mood disorder and into the light in a captivating, enlightening way.

> **Professor Gordon Parker AO**
> *Professor of Psychiatry University of New South Wales,*
> *and psychiatrist Black Dog Institute.*

I had three children and imagined I knew most things about having a baby. I didn't. Jen Wight's story made my hair stand on end. She took me through a labyrinth of happenings, from postpartum psychosis to depression. At times she imagined she was Cameron Diaz; at other times, that she would be awarded a Nobel Prize for curing cerebral palsy with dental floss. Her accounts are backed by medical explanations and are courageous and informative.

She introduces us to her partner, known affectionately as The Norwegian, who takes over feeding and cuddling their baby. Lack of sleep means the couple struggle. I think back to some of my own early difficulties, and recognise that not nearly enough has been written acknowledging the problems of early motherhood. For some women, it's a breeze; for others, it can be frightening – which is why Jen Wight's memoir, Day Six, is such a brilliant contribution to one of the most important experiences in human life, and one of the most mysterious.

> **Anne Deveson AO**
> *Author of "Tell Me I'm Here"; co-founder of Sane Australia*
> *and the Schizophrenia Fellowship of NSW;*
> *former member NSW Mental Health Tribunal*

This book is a brave and honest account of what it's really like to experience a mental illness at the very time when you are expected to be most content: when you're a new mother. It's not only a compelling read, but a moving insight into how psychiatric illness affects not only your mind, but also your body, your relationships and the sense of who you are.

Dr Dawn Barker
Psychiatrist & author of "Fractured"

In Day Six, Jen Wight has written a very important book. She charts the territory of postnatal psychosis and depression with clarity and detail, giving the reader first-hand experience of these states. Hers is a vivid, highly personal, and graphic account of a terrifying experience that we need to understand a great deal more about.

As with many female conditions, not nearly enough is known and communicated about postpartum disorder, and so each sufferer has her experience made far worse by the isolation and ignorance that attends it. Jen's book could do much to throw light on this not uncommon condition. It will be invaluable for all those close to someone going through it; and friends, partners and families needing support and enlightenment.

As a patron of the mental health charity SANE, I also think it will be of great use to mental health practitioners, and to all those midwives, nurses and doctors who are close at hand in the weeks following birth.

Jen Wight has written with great courage, vision and wit – and has produced a book of real insight and value.

Juliet Stevenson CBE
Award winning actress and patron of SANE UK

This book will give the reader a very special insight into the remarkable journey that Jen encountered. It is fascinating to read of her experiences, documented with brutal and beautiful honesty throughout. A fabulous book that I found impossible to put down.

Bibi Kennedy
Clinical nurse specialist

Jen Wight has written a book for Everywoman, and Everyman for that matter. The reader is taken on a journey with Jen as she traverses postnatal psychosis and depression and finally finds the road again.

There is humour too – I couldn't help laughing at the way Jen decides she can discover a cure for cerebral palsy using just dental floss. Yet there is a rationale for this which helps us understand, in a very intimate way, the internal reality of a mind reaching for meaning and purpose in the midst of chaos.

There is also love, care and patience, from 'The Norwegian', from Jen's parents, sister and friends, from most of the professionals she meets.

I recommend this book to all those encountering or who have encountered problems around becoming a parent, to the professionals who work with them, to researchers in the field and to everyone else as well.

Dr Fiona C Kennedy,
Consultant Clinical Psychologist, MD, GreenWood Mentors Ltd.
B.A., M. Clin Psychol., D. Clin Psych., C. Psychol., AFBPS,
BABCP Accredited Practitioner, Supervisor and Trainer

x

About The Author

Jen Wight is an author, writer, charity fundraiser and photographer.

She currently works for the Cerebral Palsy Alliance and has raised millions of dollars for social justice causes since starting her fundraising career in 2002.

Jen was the city editor for the 2009 Not for Tourists London guide (NFT) and she wrote a regular column for N16 magazine. She has contributed reviews for London, Hong Kong and Sydney to the travel website www.wcities.com; written features for Time Out Sydney, Third Sector and Wed; reviews for www.viewlondon.com, Big Screen magazine and Cornish World; travel pieces for www.expeditioner.com; and profiles for Friction Climbing magazine.

Jen hales from Hackney in east London and lives in Fairlight, Sydney with her son, husband and their imaginary dog, Fart.

Website: www.jenswight.com

Foreword

One thing that often happens to new mothers, between 50–80% of them, is what's known as the baby blues. New mothers can feel sad, over emotional and weepy at some point in that first crazy week of a baby's life. It is so common that it is considered normal, and is thought to be linked to the huge hormonal changes after birth, combined with the massive emotional upheaval of actually becoming a mother. It doesn't usually last longer than a week. Usually. In my case this period was the start of a long descent into madness and depression. And it all started on Day Six.

This story, about the first year of my son's life, is my equivalent of climbing the north face of the Eiger, being kidnapped by jungle rebels, or being wrongly imprisoned for a crime I didn't commit. Surviving the sixth day of my baby's life was the third most difficult thing I've ever done. It took all my physical and mental strength—all my coping mechanisms, all my grit and determination. The second most difficult—well that was the mind-bending events that happened in the sixth week. And the most ... is revealed in the following pages.

I was one of those new mothers without any experience of looking after a small baby. I'd never changed a nappy or settled a baby to sleep. I'd never bottle-fed one, let alone tried to breastfeed. I naively thought you couldn't take a baby outside for the first six weeks of his or her life until a kind friend told me that was kittens not babies.

What follows in this book are my recollections, as accurately as I can remember them given I was whacked out on painkillers, beside myself with sleep deprivation and blissed out on being a mother. So take them with a pinch of salt or whatever inert compound takes your fancy. I have tried to be as truthful as I can and have only made additions where it adds to the clarity of the readers' experience.

Read this book if you are thinking of having kids but are worried about mental health—either yours or someone else's.

Read this book if you've always wondered what people mean when they say having a child changes everything, but have never been able to explain how.

Read this book if having a baby was the toughest, most wonderful thing you've ever done, and have wondered why there aren't more books about the first weeks of life.

Contents

About The Author	ix
Foreword	x
Chapter One	1
Chapter Two	7
Chapter Three	11
Chapter Four	15
Chapter Five	19
Chapter Six	25
Chapter Seven	35
The Transition	37
Chapter Eight	39
The psychosis	45
Chapter Nine	47
Chapter Ten	53
Chapter Eleven	57
Chapter Twelve	63
Chapter Thirteen	69
Chapter Fourteen	79
Chapter Fifteen	85
Chapter Sixteen	89
The Hospital	93
Chapter Seventeen	95
Chapter Eighteen	99
Chapter Nineteen	113
Chapter Twenty	125
Chapter Twenty One	129
Postnatal Depression	135
Chapter Twenty Three	141
Chapter Twenty Four	145
Recovery	155
Chapter Twenty Six	157
Chapter Twenty Seven	161
Postscript	165
Support	169

Day Six

'How can a day be so hard, wonderful, thrilling, amazing, tiring, frightening, weird, cool, confusing, painful, stressful, brilliant, funny, trippy, revealing, sad, happy, fun and exciting ALL AT THE SAME TIME.'

My Diary Entry

Chapter One

Day Six begins at midnight on 2nd February. I fell asleep at 10.00 pm so I'm pretty groggy when a nurse brings me The Boy to feed. I know a lot of mums have two hours between feeds in the early days, but I've always been greatly affected by interrupted sleep. My breasts are tight and full like two over-ripe tomatoes capped with scabbed and bleeding nipples. I attach my limpet-mouthed baby on the least painful of my breasts, on the right, and settle back for the feed. I attach him to the more painful one, on the left, when the right seems empty. I wince as he somehow manages to kick my caesarean scar despite lying horizontally across my body. I wrap him tightly in the standard pale blue, yellow and pink hospital blanket and tuck him back into the bassinet. Stumbling into the startling light of the corridor, and into the cacophony of the nursery, I hand him over to one of the nurses.

This is the last of five nights at the private hospital. Private health insurance is a condition of the 457 work visa that entitles my husband and me to work in Australia for four years.

It's the best money we've ever spent. Trying to come to grips with this new, tiny, jaundice-yellow, scrap of life was made so much easier being in a private en suite room with magnificent views of Sydney. Three meals a day plus snacks helped too, with tasty home-made broths in tiny cream-coloured bowls and non-mushy veg with everything.

Having your own bathroom also really comes in handy when you're leaking large gobs of blood onto tombstone-sized sanitary towels and lying on another flat absorbent pad to catch any blood that the sanitary towel misses; not to mention the pain of the letterbox-sized wound that the baby was delivered through.

But the best thing is having a rotating cast of midwives, physios, nurses and lactation consultants in the wings. And the fact that they will look after your baby while you sleep, or in my case, try to.

When The Obstetrician came to check on me post-operation on Day One he said, 'Don't feel bad about putting the baby in the nursery every night, you catch up on sleep.' He is large and kindly with a tired smile on his lips. So I took him at his word and didn't feel bad. Much.

Watching the staff in the nursery is a good way to learn no harm comes from letting babies cry for a bit. These miniature new humans are incredibly resilient. They will not spontaneously combust, die of hunger or drown in their own tears. It's OK to cry, and yet we are consistently taught not to almost from the moment we are born.

When The Boy was born we were given a marvellous clear plastic bassinet which doubles up as a baby bath. We wheel him around going to breastfeeding classes or physio. And at night when The Boy is asleep I wheel him into the nursery. One end of each bassinet is propped up on its metal frame so the staff can easily keep an eye on their noisy charges. In the nursery the babies are wrapped tight, like Eskimo offspring, sleeping or crying in rows. Somehow, at any given time, at least half the babies manage to sleep like, well, babies.

* * *

After handing The Boy over to the nursery staff, I return to my room and pad about getting ready for sleep. I phase out for a while in a dream-like state, then I realise for the last 20 minutes I've been rearranging the items on my bedside table. This is one of those tables with wheels that you can slide over someone propped up in bed. First my eye mask, then glass of water, biscuit, mobile, and call console. The call console is TV remote-sized, and has a volume control, channel changer and a large central call button. It's attached to the wall behind the bed with a long white cable.

No, I'll need the water nearest and then the call console in the middle, so it doesn't fall off. I step back and survey the table. No, I think I'll put on the eye mask now, but just not put it over my eyes, then ...

So far so OCD. A jolt of fear goes through me. What am I doing? Trying to find the correct order? But that's crazy. The words *anxiety disorder* flash before me in looping handwriting.

* * *

Earlier the previous day, while The Boy was sleeping for long stretches, I started to worry about the medication I was on. Could it affect him? It's a tricyclic antidepressant called amitriptyline. This was one of the first antidepressants developed and over the years, doctors have discovered that at a low dose—too low to work as an antidepressant—it has a very beneficial effect on facial pain, headaches and migraines.

I had been suffering from excruciating headaches and after trying a number of different treatments including Botox, agonisingly injected into my jaw and temples, I was referred to a neurologist. He told me, what I already knew, that the headaches were caused by grinding and clamping my teeth at night. He also told me about a type of amitriptyline but, after checking my age (35 aka desperate for a baby as far as he was concerned) said, 'It is poison for babies. Poison. So you can't start a family while taking it.'

Turns out he had me pegged. I'd been preparing to try for a baby; getting all my jabs up to date and switching from the pill—which I'd been on, on-and-off, since I was 16—to condoms.

I went to see my GP and told her that, given what the neurologist had said, I had no choice but to put off trying for a baby because I really needed to try the amitriptyline. But she, the marvellous woman that she is, said,

'Let's just double check and ring MotherSafe.'

This is a wonderful free phone service run by nurses. They told me the risk was very, very low on the dose of the drug I would be taking. Did I mention it is too low a dose to work as an antidepressant? Yes? Well anyway, it is.

They did tell me to avoid a homebirth as the baby might be sleepy and need to be monitored at hospital. As I'd rather give birth through my ear than have a homebirth this was no problem. So, out went the condoms and we starting trying for a baby.

* * *

But now, with The Boy's little yellow face staying smooth with sleep for hour after hour, I start to worry. While I'm on the phone to MotherSafe, a woman comes into our room. She is in her late forties and, unlike most of the staff, not wearing a uniform. She has a stern matronly air.

'Hello.' she says, ignoring the fact that I'm on the phone.

The Norwegian says, 'We are on the phone to Mother Care.'

She looks puzzled.

'MotherSafe,' I mouth.

'Oh, yeah, MotherSafe.'

The very friendly lady on the phone is able to reassure me again and I hang up. I smile to The Norwegian.

'They don't think it should be a problem.'

'Why did you ring MotherSafe?'

I explain about the amitriptyline once I get off the phone.

'Why didn't you ask one of us?' she asks with her eyebrows drawn together. 'They just have *The Book*; really, they just read out of *The Book*. We are the ones who know about all the medication. They are going to think we don't know what we are doing. Really!' She stands over us.

'I've always found them very useful,' I say. 'I've had to explain over and over to each shift about the amitriptyline and why I'm taking it. The nurses say, 'How are the headaches, dear?' and I have to explain that I take the medication everyday prophylactically to avoid getting headaches, rather than a painkiller for the headaches. That's why.'

She purses her lips as I go on. My abdomen is throbbing and aching.

'They also keep getting the name muddled up with the painkiller I'm taking.' I was taking a strong painkiller but I'd stopped after one day because I felt so spaced out and trippy I wasn't sure which end the nappy went on and which end the milk went in. But I don't tell her that. I find out later that this painkiller is in the same family of drugs as methadone and heroin.

The Nurse leaves the room and returns a few minutes later with *The Book* as well as my notes. The Norwegian is in the bathroom. She comes to sit down opposite me. The wheelie table is inbetween us.

'This is all they read out from. Really you should have just asked one of us.' She flicks through the book and finds the drug's brand name. I don't point out to her that all she is doing is reading out from *The Book* as well. *The Book* in question is a comprehensive list of all medication and information about risks for pregnant or breastfeeding women.

'Ah,' she says. Her eyebrows unknit and eyes soften.

'You're taking antidepressants.'

'Yes.' I feel a tinge of shame. 'But my understanding is this low dose doesn't function as an antidepressant but does get rid of migraines and tension headaches. Both of which I have.'

'So you were having tension headaches?'

'Yes, I was grinding my teeth at night.'

'Why?'

Thinking about why, a wave of tiredness breaks over me. I lean over and start to cry, not full-blown tears but tired hiccups of sadness.

'I had a very stressful family situation that was unresolved for many months. I started getting excruciating headaches. I was told that I was grinding my teeth at night and this was causing the headaches.'

She reaches for a box of tissues. Gone are the harsh lines and *The Book* lies forgotten in front of her.

'Taking the amitriptyline has made all the difference. I also started seeing a counsellor and have been doing lots of yoga, that really helped too,' I say trying to sound more positive.

She murmurs some words of comfort as she flips open the red folder of my notes and reads through. She stops at one point and taps the paper with her pen. The loo flushes and I can hear The Norwegian washing his hands.

'It says here anxiety disorder.' She points at the words with her pen.

'What? Where did you get that from?'

The Norwegian comes back into the room frowning.

'The person who rang you before admission to get a background.'

The day before admission a woman had rung me to explain what I needed to do on the big day and asked me some background questions. It seems that the way I had explained my headaches had led her to believe I had an anxiety disorder. Who knows, maybe I do?

The power of IT IS IN YOUR NOTES really hits me. I'd never been told before that what I had was an anxiety disorder. All it takes is for one person to not listen to you properly, or to not be up-to-date with current medication, to put something like an anxiety disorder on your permanent record—and on your worry list.

'So, you do have an anxiety disorder.'

'But I'm not taking the amitriptyline as an antidepressant.'

'Nevertheless.'

She closes my notes and asks about breastfeeding. I explain about all the difficulties I've been having and she promises to send in one of the lactation consultants.

When she leaves I burst into proper tears and The Norwegian hugs me.

'God, I've got an anxiety disorder.'

'No, Jen, that is just what someone thought after speaking to you for five minutes.'
'But maybe I do.'
'I don't think you do.'
'I'm so tired,' I say.

* * *

Later that night The Norwegian is sparked out on the bed, The Boy is asleep again and the TV burbles in the background. I'm tidying up the room walking around with my breasts out. Because the room is actually quite chilly, thanks to the air conditioning, I have a wrap around top that I've tied underneath my breasts to give them a good airing. This is to help them heal. I look like a bloated, kinky ballerina. I walk past the dark window and catch something out of the corner of my eye. I freeze. On one of the balconies in the building opposite there is the dark shadow of a man with binoculars focused on my window. I rush to the window to close the shutters. I sit on the chair, breathing fast. I think about waking The Norwegian. But then The Boy stirs. The Boy starts to cry and The Norwegian opens one eye looking around the room. In the flurry of activity I forget about the man on the balcony and I don't mention it to The Norwegian in the hours before he leaves and heads for home.

Chapter Two

But now, in the evening, with no Norwegian and no Boy I'm standing by the bedside table with my hands resting either side the row of objects. Something is amiss, I think, very amiss. Was someone really looking through the window earlier or was I just being paranoid? Now I appear to have anxiety disorder, paranoia *and* OCD. My mental state is in a state. I abandon the sorting and climb into bed pulling the table over so I can reach the water and the call console. I feel the fear coursing through me. *Calm down*, I say to myself, *calm down*.

I lie on the bed, mask over my eyes, and pull the blankets up to my chin. I know I must sleep. I'm so tired, but my thoughts are racing, tumbling over themselves. Maybe this is it. This is when it finally happens to me. My heart is beating fast in my chest. My conscious tries to catch up with my unconscious. *Something is seriously amiss*, I think again. The panic rises in a cold tide from my stomach. *Right*, I say to myself. *Right, you are in a bad situation, things are tough but you have options, remember. Deep breath. Good. And then another.* Slowly I get my breathing under control though my heart is still pounding.

It is 1.17 am.

First, I try The Norwegian's method of going to sleep; to daydream. I have written a bestselling book—this one you are holding—and I donate half a million pounds to the wonderful charity I used to work for in east London, Quaker Social Action. I picture the moment I tell Judith, the CEO, that I'm giving them a donation. She and the board can spend it on whatever they want. Tears prickle my eyes as I imagine how pleased Judith would be, and the difference the organisation would make to the lives of people in east London living with poverty.

But I start worrying about all the people, suddenly remembering an old friendship, calling up and asking me for a donation or loan. So I imagine, then, that I will set up a grant-giving foundation. I imagine the logo, and who would be on the board. I imagine that I'll give donations only to pay for fundraisers' salaries, and janitors, and new toilets, and all the other things that most funders won't touch. God, that would be so great ... that would be

… I sigh, opening my eyes. This isn't working.

It is 1.56 am.

Maybe TV will do the trick. I pick up the console and flick on the TV and scan through the channels. I start watching a budget version of *Alien*. The alien is a disgusting hybrid-being with rows of slime-covered teeth and vicious mechanical arms. It is stalking the humans on a spaceship and as it leaps out ripping limbs from bodies, the TV screen ripples and the alien jumps out at me. I feel the fear again. Huge and overwhelming. I grab the console to change the channel. I look at the call button, should I call for help? Am I in trouble? My thumb hovers over the big square button. No. I'm fine. Really … I trace the square button with my thumb. I can't do it. Instead I start flipping through the channels again.

I settle on an early episode of *Charmed*. The actresses look fresh-faced and the film quality is a bit blurry. Most probably the first season. Lame but harmless, I think. But lame it is not—after five minutes I am gripped by the story of a tiny baby needing to be saved by the *Charmed* Ones. The dialogue is top notch; acting BAFTA-award winning. Surely it can't be that good a small voice whispers in my ear. Surely … but then the one from *90210* nearly gets killed and I am swept along by the story again. First seasons are almost always the best anyway. As the end credits scroll down the screen I sigh and get up to go to the toilet. I grab a chocolate biscuit and a swig of water before I inch myself back to bed.

It is 2.34 am.

Another program has started: *Absolutely Fabulous*. If I thought *Charmed* was good, then this, this is the best program I have ever seen. I've always thought it was good but it transcends all other comedy I've ever seen before. It makes me laugh so hard I have to press my hand over my caesarean scar for fear of busting a stitch. Saffy is having a baby and Eddie is useless, Patsy jealous. I laugh and laugh until tears run down my face. I can't wait for tomorrow when I can order a box set online. I text my parents back in London saying all is well; it's their daytime.

As the theme music comes to an end my bubbling high flips down and I am suddenly choked with fear again. Both programs featured new babies—a bit of a coincidence, I think. It is too weird. *Charmed* isn't that good, what's going on? Is this madness? Is it happening to me at last? I sit up in bed, marooned in the centre of the room. I feel the miles between me and The

Norwegian asleep at home. I feel so far from home it makes me dizzy—my parents and sisters are thousands of miles away and the gulf is yawning around me.

Is this what going insane is like? The darkness swirls around the room, almost like a living thing.

Am I on the slippery slope towards mental illness?

I cry. And then sob. *Come on Jen don't give up; there must be something else you can try?* Yoga, I think. Yoga. I relax my feet, my feet are relaxed, I relax my calves, my calves are relaxed. I relax my knees … but my monkey mind jumps. God, what is happening to me? I'm so tired but I can't sleep. I'm up, then I'm down. I must sleep; I must sleep. I push the eye mask up and check the time.

It is 2.59 am.

I try some mindfulness. *This too shall pass,* I say, *this too shall pass.* What shall pass? I think. Madness? If I'm mad then I need to ask for help. Am I going mad, is this it? How can I be so happy and laughing, then so sad all at once? Manic depression, perhaps? I start crying in earnest now. Paranoia and doubt wrap their arms about me in the dim light. I remember The Nurse waving my notes at me and tapping them with her pen. 'You have an anxiety disorder!' Down. Down. Down.

It is 3.15 am.

I think about ringing my parents but the vision of them being so distressed on learning I have gone mad breaks a huge wave of sadness over me, again and again. I can't go mad; it'll kill my parents. Well then what should I do? Push the button. But I'm scared. You've nothing to fear but fear itself. Feel the fear, and do it anyway, just do it.

Oh, God, I'm using advertising slogans to cope with this. I must be going mad. Push the button. A Chemical Brothers' song goes round my head. Dur dur da. The time has come to PUSH THE BUTTON. Dur dur da. I love the Chemical Brothers; I must buy tickets to see them play.

AM

Oh, God, I must be going mad if I'm thinking about buying gig tickets. The tears are streaming down my face. All my arguments come around to this one thought: what am I going to do? Keep making decisions like *Touching the Void* Simpson. He nearly died, but he didn't die. All roads lead back to this. Every decision is a good decision.

GOING

I've used every trick, every single thing I know to calm myself down, every self-soothing activity, and nothing has worked. I sit with the console in my hand with my finger over the button. The call button is the largest button on the console, square with rounded corners glowing green in the dark. It should say DONT PANIC like *The Hitchhiker's Guide to the Galaxy*. Where is Douglas Adams when you need him? I sob. Oh, God. I touch my hands to my swollen face and rock backwards and forwards.

MAD

The bed I'm sitting in is a rocket ship about to be blasted into space. In my ears the countdown rings out like the *Thunderbirds* theme tune.

FIVE – This is ridiculous I laugh.

FOUR – I'm laughing while I'm going mad—so I must be mad.

THREE – Or maybe I really am in a space rocket.

TWO – I know I'm not in a space rocket. I need help. I must press the button.

ONE.

BLAST OFF.

Finally, finally, finally my face ablaze with tears I push the button.

Chapter Three

The door opens and a dark figure is outlined in the bright light of the corridor. I can hear two nurses chatting softly at the nurses' station just outside my room and the bing-bing-bing of another room bell going.

'Yes, love,' says The Nurse. She stands tall with arms folded leaning against the doorframe. Her hair is dark and cut short. It glows, backlit by the fluoro light of the corridor. As my eyes adjust I can see she has a kind face, deeply lined in the way only years in the Australian sun can produce.

'I'm having a really hard ...' I sob still clutching the call console. She comes into the room and gently closes the door.

'Can you tell me what is wrong?'

I pause trying to collect myself. Just say it, Jen; just say it. SAY IT.

'I think, I really think that I'm going ... mad.' The word hangs in the air as The Nurse looks at me. I rush on:

'I'm happy and sad at the same time. I'm frightened so frightened. I thought someone was staring at me through the window. It's all so weird. I thought *Charmed* was really good when I've always thought it is quite a shit program ...'

She interrupts me. 'Don't worry. This is all totally normal.'

'Normal?'

'Yes, almost all women go through this at around about three days after their babies are born. It's the baby blues. You're exhausted.'

'Yes.'

'And your hormones are plummeting.'

'But, I really think ...'

'It happened with me, too, when I had my babies. Long before I started working here. And almost every day in my work here I see women really upset, happy and sad, and having such strange experiences.'

'It happened with you?'

The fear loosens its grip and I stare at her in wonder. This is normal? I think: I'm not going mad. My biggest fear, the one that has dogged me all my life, my very worst fear, isn't coming true. She is my saviour in a pale green tunic, my small-hours guardian angel. Relief floods through me.

As I was to find out later, many women experience what is known as 'baby blues' around day three or four when all the hormones that have built up over the nine months of pregnancy, combined with the sheer mind blowing head-mess of actually becoming a parent, causes some very wobbly behaviour.

In her bible for Australian mums, *Baby Love*, the parenting guru Robin Barker says: 'As many as 70% of women experience the baby blues. They are strongly associated with hormone imbalance. Occasionally baby blues can be prolonged and traumatic and herald the onset of major depression, but some women find they are a much-needed emotional release.'

* * *

'I can assure you that is it totally normal,' The Nurse says. 'I know that doesn't make it any easier, does it?

The best thing to do is have a good cry; turn the sound up on the TV if you are worried about someone hearing you, and just have a good old cry.'

'Are you sure I'm not going mad? I thought the bed was a rocket ship.'

'Yes, really—you are just tired, love.'

'Thank you so much. Really, really.'

'My pleasure. Honestly, just let it all out.'

She closes the door behind her. I sit up on the bed with a box of tissues in front of me and let rip. I cry and cry. My face oozes sadness from my eyes, nose and mouth. I sob and heave and cry thinking of my parents, my sister, and all the pain. I think about the months of misery with my headaches. All the pain and hurt I have felt since I was 15 comes flooding out, literally dripping down my face and into the steadily growing mound of tissues. I cry and cry for hours, tears washing my face clean. Finally, at around 5.00 am, I slip into exhausted unconsciousness, surrounded by a drift of tissues.

* * *

A few years ago The Norwegian and I were staying with my parents for the Easter weekend. On Sunday night, my mum dug up a load of old photos to show my other half, childhood holidays mainly—the photos charting the change from toddler to child, child to teenager.

Three photos got me.

One was of my sister and me holding hands when she was six and I was three, wearing our matching stripy t-shirt dresses. The other two were of my sister and me on holiday in Cyprus. I was 14, she was 17. In one photograph we are lying on a bright white sandy beach asleep with our heads almost touching on a crumpled beach towel. In the other photograph she has her arm around my shoulders and is gazing at the camera. I am looking up at her, adoringly. She is so beautiful and calm, with a Mona Lisa smile.

As my mum handed the photos to me she said, 'You two always did love each other so much.'

This was the last family holiday we had before my sister suffered a severe breakdown and was caught in the jaws of schizophrenia. That was 22 years ago. She was sectioned, taken from our family home and, for many months, locked into the local psychiatric unit, in her first of many hospital stays. The day she was admitted to hospital was 15th March, Red Nose Day, and I can remember our English teacher dressed as a clown when all I could think about was my sister vomiting in the bath, and then Mum calling our GP. When I came home that night my parents told me she had been admitted to Homerton Hospital psychiatric unit. I was 15 and she was 18.

For the first few weeks my sister slept in a corridor divided up into 'bedrooms' by heavy green and brown curtains. She was locked in with people whom I, a fairly hardy Hackney girl, would have crossed roads to avoid. Shouters, screamers, silent rockers. All confused, drugged and unhappy.

So on that Easter Sunday, looking at those photos, my feelings took a nostalgia trip and grief and pain returned for the evening. That Easter I slipped into the grief again like it was a comfortable old jumper. I'd forgotten the feeling of crying quietly lying on my back in bed with the tears falling sideways and filling up my ears. I remember thinking all those years ago that my beautiful sister would act this way because she had died and something else was moving her leaden, drugged body around, making it do and say horrible things. I can remember thinking that, but I had forgotten how it felt.

I had forgotten how easy being unhappy all the time had felt.

Chapter Four

I am roused from deep, deep sleep for The Boy's next feed. It is 5.55 am. The nurse bringing the baby in is cheery and doesn't bat an eyelid at my wrecked face and battlefield-bed strewn with slaughtered tissues. I'm exhausted but feel light and free. It is like the years of worry about my sister, and my own fear of losing my mind, have been washed away by the flood of tears. Apart from my cracked, sore nipples, I feel amazing. I look down on my little son lying awake in his bassinet and waiting for my milk and feel a surge of happiness and contentment.

* * *

When I was a teenager, I was absolutely convinced that I would go mad like my sister. Every year on 15th March I would wait for the cloak of madness to descend. Three years to the day when I was 18, and in my first year at university, I spent the entire day in bed. I waited all day, not worrying about my studies, just waiting and crying. But when the day passed with no voices ringing in my ears or strange hallucinations jumping around my room, rather than feeling relieved, I readjusted my imagined fate to the following year. As I got older I realised this was like one of those cults who predict the end of the world, and then when the allotted day passes, quickly recalculate.

* * *

As the years have passed the fear has diminished and now, after my night of terror, I realise that if I can survive a night like that without going mad, then I can survive anything. Little do I know the terror of the night before will pale into insignificance by the mind-bending experience of Week Six.

* * *

I clear away the tissues and prepare myself, lining up a glass of water and another biscuit to keep me going until breakfast. I send The Norwegian a text saying all is going well and that he doesn't need to rush in.

When I half open the shutters and check out the building opposite, I find the balcony where I saw the man with the binoculars actually has a large human shaped plant in a pot on it. I laugh and pull the shutters fully open.

The feeling of contentment swells and I bring my son to my breast and he latches on the first time.

* * *

This is quite an achievement. 'The latch' is the holy grail of breastfeeding and I've been struggling with it right from the start. The very first feed was only a few hours after my operation when I still couldn't move my legs after the epidural. One of the nurses helped me with the latch.

The Boy was a determined feeder from the beginning and sucked with all his might.

The Nurse—one of the few I didn't like—asked,

'Does it hurt?'

You are supposed to feel a few toe-curling seconds of pain which should fade away if the latch is done correctly.

'Well no,' I said, 'but given that I can't feel my legs, or the gash in my abdomen the baby came out of, I should think nothing would hurt me now.'

'Good, then the latch is OK,' she said as she marched out.

Twenty minutes later when she returns she closely inspects my breast.

'Oh there is a blister, you must have not latched him on properly.'

'Must I not?'

The blister on one side soon developed into a crack, closely followed by a crack on the other. Now I was the non-proud owner of two scabbed nipples almost as painful to look at as to touch.

* * *

Breastfeeding is truly a biological marvel and I was determined give my son the best breastmilk known to man. As well as the amitriptyline, I'd also taken anti-nausea medication for the first 18 weeks of pregnancy due to extreme sickness, and add to that an elective caesarean, I was determined to at least 'do this right'. I'd learnt at my antenatal classes that your breasts will provide milk when they are stimulated by a baby feeding, the more stimulation the nipples get the sooner your milk will 'come in'.

The first few latches are vital as this is when breasts produce colostrum, rich in nutrients and antibodies. Also, the nurses know they must start teaching the mother and baby to get the latch right from the start to avoid getting into bad habits. The focus is very much on the latch rather than getting the monsters off your breast at the end of a feed, which was my problem.

The advice given in hospital is to always break the suction of the baby's mouth by 'gently inserting a finger into the corner of his mouth and then disengaging'. Most babies, I found out afterwards, will stop sucking after they have had enough milk, or just when they feel like it. I know other women who have had the opposite problem to me with their babies not sucking for long enough to stimulate the breast.

The Boy, by contrast, is what is called a voracious feeder, sucking and sucking long after any early milk was delivered into his hungry stomach. If you have ever seen a YouTube video of a terrier holding onto a stick with stubborn ferocity while being spun around, then you will have a good idea of the grip my son has during breastfeeding.

To unlatch The Boy I have to insert my finger and prise open his jaw, and only then remove my flat nipple from his mouth. By the way, a flattened nipple is another sign of an incorrect latch. But I don't learn that until I am out of the hospital.

* * *

This morning I have one breast too sore to use and, after feeding for five minutes, the pain is beyond toe-curling in the other. I try to release The Boy's mouth using a gentle digit. He clamps down on my nipple and tears the scab away. My once beautiful breast starts to bleed. Now neither of my nipples are working as a dispenser of breakfast. I hold the baby away from my body as his face crunches into the cry of a newborn—like a lamb bleating down a tin-can telephone. My calm elation gets up and flies out the window as his cries increase in volume.

I reach for the console and this time press the button without hesitation. I hum 'der der dum', the time has come to PUSH THE BUTTON and the ghost of the fear I felt the night before peeps over my shoulder. But then the door opens and the lifesaver sweeps into the room.

This Nurse is English with glossy black skin, a bosom you could balance a tray on and an English cut glass, home-counties accent. She saw me through my second night, helping me learn the latch with patience, reminiscing about England and Sainsbury's sausages. I remember the contrast of my glowing white breasts and her dark hands as she patiently helped me practise the swooping movement of a tried and tested latch.

'Thank God it's you.' I explain what has happened.

'I think I'm too sore to carry on breastfeeding.'

She examines my chest with a practised eye.

'These need a rest. I'll get some formula. And the form.' She rolls her eyes at me and she pulls the door shut behind her. I walk around the room jiggling The Boy as his cries build and build. The form, as it turns out, is a waiver I have to sign before I can get the formula. I have to sign that I am aware that using formula could negatively affect my ability to breastfeed in the future. It is just formula, not formaldehyde, but I imagine a lawyer somewhere has worked out the hospital may get sued by a frantic mother who blames the nurses for using formula, when the mother was at a low ebb. Or maybe they already have.

'I'm sorry about the form but we really have to get it signed.'

'I don't mind. There's no way I could do more breastfeeding right now.'

'We'll make sure you have someone show you how to express so you can rest your nipples.' I imagine my nipples going off to a rest home for battered body parts as she shows me how to hold The Boy and bottle-feed. Peace descends on the room once more.

'See, you're a natural,' she says as she glides from the room like a galleon in full sail. As she leaves there is a knock at the door. The first of many. It is breakfast.

'Lovely morning,' I say to the orderly as he places the tray on my table. He looks everywhere but at me and, as he closes the door behind him, I realise I've tied my wrap under my breasts again and my battered beauties are on display. And I just don't care.

Chapter Five

I'm tucking into my breakfast of cornflakes, tea and toast, with The Boy cooing in his bassinet as The Norwegian arrives.

It is 7.34 am.

'Had to start him on formula as my boobs are wrecked,' I say. 'I've had such a strange, awful night, really weird.'

The Norwegian constructs a bacon sandwich from my leftovers as I finish my tea.

'What happened? Was it The Boy?'

'He was in the nursery, but still I only had about two hours of sleep, and I'm knackered.

'Two hours? Why?'

The door opens and a kindly lady with a face full of wrinkles and a sweep of white hair steps in.

'FLOWERS,' she bellows at the top of her voice.

The flower ladies are all volunteers at the hospital making sure any flowers are well looked after. She looks around the room.

'Ah still no flowers,' she says looking at me. Her wrinkles have rearranged themselves into a map of concern.

We smile at her and I say,

'Nope no flowers,' and she pulls the door shut behind her.

On our first day she'd shouted FLOWERS and looked around the room for any trace of a pale petal or glossy leaf. In her world no flowers, when you've just had a baby, is like an elephant without a trunk. It just isn't right. Almost as if flowers are an essential part of the birthing process, perhaps delivered by the mother in between the baby and the placenta.

'I should have just bought some flowers,' says The Norwegian. 'Just to keep her happy. Do you remember we went in the lift up the maternity ward with her?'

'Oh, yes!' I say.

She had vicious looking shears and secateurs laid out like surgical instruments on a metal trolley. *I hope she doesn't do your delivery* The Norwegian had whispered to me.

'So what happened last night?' The Norwegian asks.

'After you went ...'

There is another knock at the door. The Obstetrician enters the room. After the greetings and hellos he says,

'Lets check your wound then.' I roll onto the bed and inch my tracksuit bottoms and knickers down. The wound glares up at him red and angry looking, fringed by pubic stubble.

The most pain I experienced on Day One, the day of the operation, was when one of the nurses shaved the top inch of my pubic hair triangle. This was more painful than the cannula being inserted into the back of my hand, the epidural injection into my spine and way more painful than the careful slicing of six layers of tissue to break into my womb.

I'd heard of women getting the whole area waxed and thought this was due to vanity or shyness about showing a room full of people their muff. I'd thought, well, the doctors and nurses will see more vaginas in one week than most people see in a lifetime. They're not going to bat an eyelid if I have hair down there. But, even though I knew the cut would be under my bikini line, I hadn't put two and two together and dealt with it myself.

'Do you have pubic hair?' The Nurse had asked me an hour before the operation was due.

'Yes,' I said thinking, well ye-es, since I'm over 14 and have managed to get myself pregnant I think you can safely say I have passed through the trials and tribulations of puberty. When she started shaving me it seemed to go on for hours as she scraped, scraped, and scraped with a razor so blunt it would make a banana look like a deadly weapon.

The Norwegian sat squirming in the corner of the room throwing me looks of mouth-twisting sympathy. Despite how long she took, she had somehow managed not to do a clean shave but left a rash of angry stubble that was to cause me some pain later when the dressings were removed.

* * *

While she scraped my hair away I pondered the subjective nature of pain. I think my jittery nervous state made the pain of my skin being dragged along under the blunt blade much worse.

* * *

But that was on day one, back in the room with The Obstetrician, he closely studies my wound and then looks up at me.

'Good. Good,' he says.

Another face with short fair hair and pale eyes pops around the door and sees the doctor.

'Oh I'll come back later,' she says shutting the door.

'Thank you, Doctor, for everything,' I say.

He smiles as I hitch up my trousers. We all look at The Boy asleep in his bassinet. The Obstetrician is speaking but I can't stop staring at the little monkey-faced baby who is actually mine. I still can't believe it. We actually have a baby.

'Intercourse,' says The Obstetrician.

'Er?' I say.

'This is going to sound strange but I have to let you know that you can still get pregnant if you have unprotected sex. It doesn't matter that your periods haven't started again. It is really important you know this.'

'Sex?' I say. With a barely healed slash inches away from my foof, and tits like unripe rock melons and a tiny newborn to look after, I can't think of a time when I have less felt like having sex. Well, apart from one of the worst bouts of cystitis I'd ever had while on a camping holiday in Wales.

I look at The Norwegian.

'Sorry darling, I don't think I'm quite in the mood.'

'Fine by me,' he says.

The doctor laughs and says, 'I bet that's the first time that's happened.'

He looks at me smiling and in a radical topic jump asks:

'How is the constipation?'

'Oh, much better thanks. I did a poo yesterday.'

You really don't mind discussing your poo with a man who has cut you open, reached in and pulled out your newest family member.

The day before, the doctor had advised me to take anti-constipation medication as I still hadn't 'opened my bowels'. Also, a women sitting next to me at a settling class in the hospital had whispered hoarsely into my ear, 'Make sure you don't get constipated. It's agony. Drink lots of water.'

*   *   *

Constipation is the enemy of pregnant women and new mothers. When I was pregnant I had been taking medication to help with extreme morning sickness and this made me constipated. I'd fire out little painful rabbit-poo-sized pellets into the bowl.

In between kneeling on the bathroom floor with my arm draped over the toilet seat, vowing to start a campaign to abolish the term morning sickness, and trying not to get caught in the splash-back following a particularly violent burst, I'd also found the time to ring The Obstetrician.

'I can't push the baby out, can I?'

'No,' he'd told me, 'But get yourself some—' and he named a well-known brand of fibre supplement.

The supplement got things moving admirably. You mix the orange powder with water and drink it quickly before it has a chance to solidify. But I did find it very disconcerting one day when I threw up an oesophagus-shaped blob of orange goo. Ah, the joys of pregnancy.

*   *   *

Back in the hospital The Obstetrician kisses my cheek and shakes The Norwegian's hand as he leaves us.

'Can you imagine having sex now?' I say. The Norwegian laughs and gives me a careful hug.

'So, tell me about last night.'

'I need a shower before the next person comes in. We need to check out by 10.00 am.'

I relax in the shower with the hot water streaming over me and the steam clouding the room. I can hear the door again and The Norwegian saying, 'She's in the shower.' I dry myself carefully dabbing at my wound and scabbed nipples to make sure they are dry. I pop my head around the door.

'All clear?' I say. The Norwegian nods.

Getting dressed I carefully pack away my battered breasts into my black maternity bra tucking a reusable breast pad into each cup. The Norwegian has started clearing the room, carefully and systematically packing my clothes and The Boy's things into a bag. In our relationship The Norwegian, with his slightly OCD tendencies, is the packer. I found out later that he'd spent a couple of hours the night before using a tape measure to measure all the onsies we had and then sorting them by size. It seemed like a perfectly sensible thing for him to do at the time.

The door goes again. It is the bright-faced, wonderful Nurse. She has shiny brown hair and a round smiley face.

'How's it going?' she says.

I tell her about my trials with breastfeeding and needing to learn how to express.

'I'll go get a machine.' Moments later she is back pushing a creamy yellow coloured machine on wheels. It has two clear plastic tubes snaking out the top and two dials on the front. She also has, what looks like, the contents of her Tupperware drawer.

'It's fairly easy once you get the hang of it,' she says as I unpack my boobs again and get ready to hook myself up to the machine. The scab on one nipple sticks to the breast pad and, as I peel it away, I rip of the scab and wince.

The Nurse says, 'Ouch. You can put a little dab of nipple cream on your nipple before you put on your bra and the scabs won't stick.'

'Next time.'

There is a knock on the door.

'Water?' says the attendant while The Nurse stands to shield me from his gaze. We'd been very confused by the water attendant as we just got tap water from the bathroom.

The Nurse patiently explains how the machine works and I give it a go. It has two speeds, one to stimulate the let down, which gets the breasts starting to work, and a faster speed to actually pump the milk out. At the end of one of the plastic tubes The Nurse attaches a funnel and a clear plastic bottle. She shows me how to attach the funnel to my breast with the nipple in the middle of the tube. Once the faster speed starts, my nipple is sucked into the tube making a pink cylinder of flesh and the flared cup of the funnel is stuck onto the surrounding breast.

'You can adjust the power here,' she shows me. 'And the idea is to have it just below the painful point.'

'My nipples are quite painful all the time,' I say.

'Ah, OK, then we will have it on a low pressure to start with.'

I can see little spurts of milk shooting out of invisible holes in my nipple and trickling down into the plastic bottle. One of the more painful things that can go wrong when you are learning to breastfeed is mastitis. Luckily, this fate didn't befall me but many women get mastitis at some point, and it is usually caused by a blocked milk duct. When you are first learning to breastfeed you're taught to massage your breast and watch for lumps; these are early warning signs of a blocked duct.

'You can hire these machines from your local chemist,' she tells us.

'You all right for now?' she asks. 'I'll be back when you've finished this to take out your stitches.'

When she has gone The Norwegian looks at me.

'I'm a human cow,' I say and he laughs as we hear yet another knock on the door.

Chapter Six

It is 8.57 am. The door opens and a tall athletically-built woman with short fair hair and pale green eyes strides in.

'Good morning. I'm one of the lactation consultants.' She stands looking at me as I am attached to the pumping machine.

'So I understand you are having trouble breastfeeding,' she says looking at the folder with The Boy's notes giving details of nappies and feeds, which we've been filling in religiously.

'I've had to stop altogether this morning as my nipples are in a terrible state.'

'Were you having problems with the latch? I see from your notes you've had a couple of the experienced nurses to help you. They are usually really good at teaching people the latch.'

'Yes, they were great, but he just sucks and sucks. Whenever I ask for someone to watch the latch they say it's fine, but by the end my nipple's even sorer and is squashed flat.'

'Maybe he was slipping off your nipple during the feed?'

'Maybe.'

'You need to reattach if that happens.'

'How can I tell?'

'Because it hurts'.

'But it hurts all the time.'

'Ah, well, it hurts more.' She falls silent as The Boy wakes and starts protesting. The Norwegian picks him up and starts walking around the room in the centuries old jigglewalk that all mothers and most fathers are arm-achingly familiar with.

'Anyway, I can tell you about formula feeding while you rest your breasts, and then you can get back to breastfeeding in a few days.'

'OK.'

* * *

I'd heard about the Breastapo but hadn't encountered a member yet. These are midwives and nurses whose keenness on breastfeeding somewhat overwhelms their ability to be kind and considerate. The lactation consultant was the closest I'd come to Breastapo, she just assumed that I would go back to breastfeeding. I was so convinced that I would breastfeed, had wanted it so badly, that it was easy to go along with her.

'So first you need to work out the dose which is the amount of formula that the baby needs.' I drift off for a second. Then it seems like she is saying, 'This is baby's weight times by his weeks of age. Then add your birthday, your weight, pi and then Planck's constant. If the month has a 'u' in it then you need to double the number you first thought of and then highflip the dingkerton squash-a-squiggy. Then you klingfarf the first feed of the day. It is really important that you remember to toddlewhap-burger the highflip … and never forget to maintain good bottle hygiene.'

'Sorry I'm finding this really hard to follow. I didn't get much sleep last night. Can you write it down?' I ask The Norwegian.

She goes on explaining and The Norwegian frowns with concentration scribbling in his notebook. I turn off the breast pump and gently break the suction to remove my poor breast from the funnel.

'I can see you've got the hang of the breast pump, anyway.'

'Yes.'

She turns to The Norwegian. 'So you see it's really quite simple,' she says as she leaves the room.

'Did you get any of that?'

'Some,' says The Norwegian frowning at the notebook in his hand.

I shake the bottle to see how much I'd managed to express. A small amount of the precious white liquid sloshes around in the bottom.

'I really want to breastfeed,' I say and I start crying and The Norwegian comes over and folds me into his arms.

'You will, you will,' he says.

The Nurse knocks and pops her head around the door.

'Oh, sorry.'

'I'm just so tired,' I say blowing my nose.

'I was going to take your stitches out. Shall I come back?' She gives us a sympathetic upside down smile.

'No, now is fine.' I hop back onto the bed and roll my trousers down again.

'I see some of your hair has grown back,' she says. She is not wrong. The dressing around the stitches is stuck to the short hairs around the wound. She inches the dressing off and I wince as it pulls and drags against the wound and surrounding puckered flesh. Then she cuts the blue thread and gently eases it out of the scabbed and red skin.

'Sorry about this,' she says.

'That's OK,' I say.

It is 10.29 am.

* * *

I'd had an elective caesarean. The Boy had been breach for most of the latter half of the pregnancy and, given the size of his head (97 percentile) and broad shoulders, The Obstetrician recommended a C-section. He said getting the body out, and then getting the head stuck, was a situation we really wanted to avoid.

'Yeah,' I laughed. 'Ouch!'

'It's not so much that,' he replied. 'The baby will have an increased chance of death or cerebral palsy.'

'I'll go for the caesarean in that case,' I said, all laughter gone from my voice.

As it turned out the caesarean went without a hitch and the birth itself lasted no more than three minutes; the whole procedure was less than an hour. The pain was non-existent, but there were some bizarre occurrences.

I was lying in the anteroom of the theatre waiting for my turn. The room was small, but fitted the large hospital bed comfortably, and had white cupboards lining one wall. The Norwegian and I had just been laughing that the sign on one of the cupboard doors had a list of contents including cocaine.

'Cut me up a line,' I said to The Norwegian in my best Ray Winston accent.

The doors to the theatre had porthole-type windows and through one I could see the infra-red lamps on the ceiling. Reflected in the round redness of one of them I could see a neat and tidy lady garden. I was just about to say to The Norwegian, 'Oh, look, I can see ...' when a scalpel hove into view and started cutting. I turned my head and buried it in The Norwegian's arm.

'What is it?'

'I can see a scalpel cutting!'

'Can we go with the stork option?' he asked.

When it was my turn they sat me up on the bed leaning forward on my bump with The Norwegian gripping both hands. I was so giddy with nerves and weirdness and the drugs they had me on, that I barely felt the injection going into my spine. I lay back with my lower half shielded from view by green sheets. The surgeons chatted about golf while they sliced me open.

'It is like being wrapped in snow,' I said to anyone who was listening to me.

'You OK?' asked The Norwegian.

I could feel them reaching in for the baby.

'It is like I am a handbag and they are reaching around for their lost keys.' We both giggled. As The Boy was being pulled out The Nurse said to The Norwegian,

'Camera time!'

As they carefully sutured the layers of flesh that made up my abdomen I could hear two nurses counting the instruments to make sure none had been left inside me.

'They sound like the improbability drive of the Heart of Gold counting down to normality,' I said. One of the reasons I love The Norwegian is that he knew exactly what I was talking about.

* * *

But back to Day Six. It is 11.03 am. There is another knock and the paediatrician comes in. She is a young Asian doctor with straight black hair and wide intelligent eyes. She lays The Boy on the bed and starts to check him over, listening carefully to his chest and gently rotating his legs.

'All OK,' she says and The Norwegian and I simultaneously let out our held breath.

'Great,' says The Norwegian.

'So you had an elective caesar,' she asks. 'Why was that?'

I told her about what The Obstetrician had said about the size of The Boy's head and shoulders and the increased risk of something going wrong at the birth. 'As it turns out,' I say, 'he wasn't as big as the scans suggested, but his head is in the 97 percentile.'

'Yes, he does have a large head.'
We all laugh and she looks up at us.
'Well, you both have large heads so it makes sense.'
I catch The Norwegian's eye but have to look away quickly.

After the blur of visitors and door-knocks we are finally ready to leave. The Norwegian goes down to bring the car around to the entrance and I wait in the nursery with our tiny little one in the bassinet. A grandpa and grandma are sitting cooing over an even tinier baby, fresh from the egg.

'Congratulations,' I say.

'Our new grandson,' says the woman, her eyes bright with tears. 'His mother is in recovery.'

The Norwegian tells me he also waited in this room with The Boy, less than a few hours old, waiting for me to come up from recovery. One of the nurses gave him tea and biscuits. He said it was the strangest hour of his life sitting waiting, in his blue scrubs and label saying DAD, with the barely born-being.

* * *

I feel a spangle-bright spark of fearlove for The Boy and pick him up for a cuddle when the text comes.

Ready.

I put The Boy back into the bassinet and wheel him out of the nursery past the nurses' station.

'We're off then,' I say.

'Great,' says one of the ladies behind the counter.

'Good luck,' says the other.

'Could you say thank you to the nurses.'

'That's lovely. Will do.'

I stand in silence looking at them.

They look back at me.

'So can I just go?'

'Yes, your husband has taken care of everything.'

'I can just take him?'

They both laugh. 'Yes love.'

I can't believe they are just going to let us take the baby. Us and a baby.

US. AND A BABY.

I feel like I'm surrounded by a force field that warps the corridor as we walk down to the lifts. I hum The Police's 'Walking on the Moon'. Dant da narrrr. The walls pulse and shimmer as if through a heat haze.

Down at the car The Norwegian slips The Boy into the car seat. I'm inside helping.

'His first drive,' I say.

'His first everything today,' says The Norwegian as he sets off. The force field is still surrounding us but it doesn't keep the cars away.

'They are so *close*. *So fast*,' I say. The Norwegian says nothing focusing all his attention on the road ahead. Cars seem to swerve and race past. The roar of traffic seems deafening. I remember a friend saying when he and his wife brought their daughter home he felt like reaching out and pushing all the other cars away.

It is a bright and sunny day. Everything seems brand new, freshly minted. The shop windows along Military Road twinkle as if just polished. I catch The Norwegian's eye in the rear-view mirror.

'Everything is so ... different,' I say.

He nods then refocuses on the road. The Boy starts a hiccuping bleat and my heart lurches. Now we have to deal with him on our own, with no help. How are we going to cope? How am I going to cope. I give him my thumb to grip and the bleats subside.

When we arrive home we find two builders working on the awning outside our front door. The Norwegian had warned me this was likely to happen. About a year and a half ago the building had some work done replacing the railings and resurfacing the walkways. At the time they had taken down the awning but never replaced it. We had been half-heartedly nagging our lovely landlady about getting it put back up, for the last year or so.

'Today of all days,' I say. 'Nice.'

The two builders greet us as we huff up the stairs.

'How you doing?' One of them asks with a strong Welsh accent. His face is all smiles, topped with wavy fair hair. He has a large tattoo on his upper arm.

'Oh fine,' says The Norwegian, 'here is our son.' He holds the carry-cot out for inspection.

'Where are you from?' I ask. 'Wales?'

'Yes, South Wales'

'Ah, him too,' I say pointing at The Norwegian. He's half Welsh—Swansea born—but having grown up in Norway is a little bit more 'Wegian than Welsh.

'I'm Donk,' he says and holds out his hand to The Norwegian.

'How funny, both from South Wales and now meeting in New South Wales.'

Donk grins even wider and I leave them to chat about rugby as I take The Boy inside.

'We'll really try to keep the noise down,' says Donk, and the other silent builder nods in agreement. And they really do. If it is possible to hammer quietly then these men—two of the most considerate builders in Australia—manage it.

It is 12.57 pm.

As we wander about the flat dazed and confused all we can hear from the outside is the dull tap tap tap as they go about fixing the problem the other builders had left behind.

I sit on the sofa with The Boy next to me in his carry-cot and The Norwegian brings me a large bowl of Shreddies. My parents had sent them over specially from the UK.

'You lucky thing,' I whisper to The Boy, 'You are going to get some Shreddie-flavoured milk. I love Shreddies and get them sent out from the UK. I once had a very vivid dream that I got one plated in gold and wore it on a chain around my neck. They are my go to breakfast cereal in all manner of situations.

I flick on the TV and *Charmed* pops up on the screen. A slight prickle makes its way down my neck. *Charmed* again? I think.

'That's weird,' I say. '*Charmed* was on the TV last night.'

The Norwegian smiles at me.

'Why weird?'

'I've got to tell you a bit about last night. I couldn't sleep and so many weird things happened.'

'Like what?'

'I really thought I was going mad. I'm so tired.'

He comes over and gives me a big hug.

'Well, why don't you tell me more about it after you've had a sleep? You need your rest. All I need to do is pop to the chemists to borrow a breast pump. Will you be all right with The Boy for 20 minutes or so?'

I look at The Boy in the carry-cot his face smooth with sleep.

'Sure.'

It is 1.34 pm.

I watch *Charmed* and am again struck with how good the program is. Really amazing. I must still be sleep-deprived, I think. I look at my watch. The Norwegian has been gone for five minutes. The Boy stirs in his cot.

Don't wake up. Don't wake up. I can't cope with you on my own. As *Charmed* plays in the background I start crying. *Why is Charmed on again? It is just too much of a coincidence.* I look at my watch. Six minutes.

Deep breathing, deep breathing. I try to slow my breath and calm myself down. My eyes flick to my watch again. Damn. Only nine minutes. I turn the TV off and start pacing the room. The tears keep bubbling up. I thought I'd got through the worst last night, but here again is the terrible fear. This is it. I'm really going mad. I sob silently not wanting the builders to hear me.

After what seems like hours The Norwegian comes back from the chemist.

'What's wrong?' he says.

'I really think I'm going mad. Really. Really. I nearly did last night. It was so awful. I couldn't press the button and ...'

'Sweetheart, you're just really tired.' He bundles me up into his arms and guides me to the bedroom.

'You just sleep now.' He is kneeling by the side of the bed, an arm around my shoulders.

'So you don't think I'm going mad?'

'No, but, Jen, no matter how many times I tell you, it doesn't matter. You need to believe it yourself.'

I relax back onto the pillow and my eyes droop.

I drop into sleep but I am still awake. My body is heavy with sleep but not my mind. My eyes are closed and my arms and legs are weighted down. But my mind won't let go. My leg jerks and I lie there waiting for my brain to switch off. My arm jerks. I will myself to sleep but my mind is blinking and beeping. It will not let go of 'awake'.

It is like I am lying submerged in water and it's lulling me to sleep but I have a small straw in my mouth that is connecting me to the awake world. This is what is must be like for babies when they are overtired. I'd heard this expression before but never understood how you could be really tired but not able to sleep.

    I can hear The Norwegian when he comes in to check on me, imagining the smile on his face when he thinks I'm asleep. My body is so heavy that I don't think I could sit up if I wanted to. The minutes stretch and yawn around me. The world whirls about my head; my single point of focus is where my body meets my mind. I feel nailed to wakefulness at this point. I wait for sleep. I wait. I wait.

Chapter Seven

I must have finally drifted off to sleep because The Boy's cries wake me up. I lie on the bed staring up at the ceiling with my breasts bursting with milk. Milk has leaked onto the sheets and my nightie. I can hear The Norwegian talking to The Boy and I drag myself up out of bed.

It is 5.45 pm.

The Norwegian hugs me as I stumble from the room.

'Did you sleep OK?'

'Sort of—it was weird.'

'That is your word of today—weird.'

'Well, it has been.'

'Are you feeling any better?'

'Yes, much,' I say turning the kettle on.

'Tea?'

'Lovely.'

The Norwegian is giving The Boy his bottle and I sit down on the sofa. The Norwegian has set up the pumping machine on the windowsill to the left of the sofa. He has also put together a feeding station with three jam jars filled with nuts and raisins, chocolate biscuits and crackers. He has filled up a large bottle of water and placed it next to a glass.

I reach over and give him a hug.

'Time to get pumping,' I say. I untie my top and carefully peel the scabbed nipples away from the breast pad. I am relieved that the scabs stay where they are. As my nipple gets rhythmically sucked in and out of the plastic tubing I try to explain what had happened the night before. The Norwegian listens in silence.

'That does sound weird.'

'See, I told you!'

By the end of pumping both breasts I've managed to express 30 ml of milk. I get up and put it in the fridge. I have a light buzzing feeling, chilled and mellow.

'I think breastfeeding is getting me high,' I say. The clever Norwegians have a phrase for it: *ammetåke* literally means breastfeeding mist.

Another to add to my vast knowledge of Norwegian words.

* * *

I have tried to pick up some Norwegian words but, partly due to the fact that most Norwegians I've met speak better English than a fair few English people, and partly because I'm monumentally awful at learning languages, my knowledge is scant at best.

I know *slobberok* (dressing-gown), *tøffler* (slippers), *øl* (beer), *tusen takk for maten* (a thousand thank yous for the meal), and of course *promp* (fart), *bæsj* (poo), and *rap* (burp). For the sake of my son's heritage it's vital that I learnt these words. I also know all the animal noises including my favourite—*vrinsk*—for a horse's neigh.

The Norwegian has defrosted one of the meals I'd made in bulk and frozen the week before The Boy was born. The table is laid with glasses of water and candles. I look at him.

'You are so wonderful,' I say.

'I know.'

We laugh.

'I love you,' I say.

'I love you too.'

'We have a baby.'

'I know.'

'US.'

'I know.'

'So weird,' I say for the final time that day.

The rest of Day Six passes uneventfully. We settle The Boy for sleep and he is sparked out by seven o'clock. We eat dinner and watch a bit of TV. We sit in bed and read before we go to sleep. We are getting the hang of things. Everything is going to be all right.

And everything *is* all right. Until Week Six.

The Transition

'Much less tired today but still not totally with it. In between pumping the right and the left boob I picked up my glass of water. Very thirsty. But instead of drinking it I offer it to my right breast. Oh dear.'

My Diary Entry

Chapter Eight

In the weeks after Day Six, the first heady weeks of The Boy's life, I am so, so happy—most of the time. The burden of 22 years' worry and fear had been rinsed from me by my marathon crying session, bringing in a tide of happiness and positivity. I love The Boy so much it feels like an explosion in my chest whenever I look at him.

This is it; now my life can begin again. It's as if a big chunk of my brain, which had been busily occupied with maintaining the draining level of fear and anxiety, suddenly finds itself with nothing to do. After a few moments of shock, it sets itself about carrying out a combination of useful new tasks: my spelling improves; I stop losing things around the apartment; I'm a better gardener and I can suddenly speak my schoolgirl French again. It also works out how to do the things I've always wanted to do—I download an app to learn Norwegian, I write my five-year life plan and I stop watching trashy TV.

I write lists and lists of the things I want to achieve, from, *find Jacky Rigby to go to every museum in Sydney,* and from *gold plate a Shreddie* to *learn taekwondo.* I plan research into internet trolls, to find out why some people are so vicious online. I think if I can find out why I might be able to stop it. I want to find out the last person to speak Latin as a proper language, and do a PhD on why Latin died out. I start planning a possible trip to Paris with my sister when The Norwegian and I are next in Europe. Since her illness I have never been away with her, even for one night, but now everything seems possible.

But as the weeks wear on the highs become higher, so much so that I write on one of my lists:

'Check with The Psychologist. Am I manic?'

And lows start appearing, with periods of extreme irritability and anxiety. Much more of a burden to The Norwegian than to me.

During my highs I have fast and furious conversations with The Norwegian about Life, the Universe and Everything (the Douglas Adams book as well as the concept). Later, he said it was like being back in college when all things felt possible—within the reach of an outstretched arm and an open mind.

We go to a friend's wedding at Long Reef Golf Club when I'm having one of my highs. The Boy sleeps in his pushchair next to the round table and chairs with big bows on the back. In between courses of lovely food, I regale the table with stories, smiling and laughing and bestowing my sparkling wonderfulness to all and sundry.

I am totally over-the-top, over loud and over bearing. I catch a few glances between some of the other guests on our table, but don't let that halt the flow of scintillating commentary I believe I am supplying.

I manage to embarrass one of the other guests, a man with red hair and a sharp wit. I've been chatting to the man next to him about his wife who is Chinese and who can't get a visa to come and live in Australia. Red joins in the conversation and I ask loudly, 'So where is your lovely wife?' He then has to announce to the table that they are separated. There is a tumbleweed moment after that, but one of the other guests manages to start the conversation again. A few minutes later, undaunted, I manage to demolish his argument as to why you shouldn't wash your hands after you've gone to the toilet.

'But they say you've got more germs under your fingernails than under the seat of the average toilet. So you should really wash the toilet seat after you've touched it with your dirty hands,' he says.

'That's why you *shouldn't* wash your hands? Because they are too dirty? Really? It's all the more reason *to* wash your hands!' I reply with a flourish beaming to all the others on our table. That'll stump him I think.

He pinches his lips together with forefinger and thumb, hiding a thwarted smile.

'Yes, that does make sense,' he says quietly while the rest of the table burst out laughing. He then avoids talking to me for the rest of the meal and between the speeches. We leave just after the dancing starts to get The Boy into his bed.

But then the lows come and I snap at The Norwegian, demanding his help with unimportant tasks, like learning how to use Pinterest, when he's exhausted from disturbed nights and trying to keep up with my racing thoughts.

And The Boy. Despite having huge problems with breastfeeding I love being a new mum, feeling full to the brim with a brand new type of love. I love learning new things, and it feels that, now I've been let into the wonderful new world of motherhood, I have the opportunity to learn 20 impossible things before breakfast. Nothing is too much for my little boy.

The times when I am most anxious usually revolve around going out. Going to my newly established mothers' group is very stressful, though I love the women I meet and am convinced they're all going to become lifelong friends.

As long as I am safe in the flat with my pumping machine, jars of snacks, cups of tea and my iPad, I'm like the happiest pig in the stinkiest of mud. I love it so much that I don't want The Norwegian to miss out and suggest he take a year's sabbatical after my maternity leave, so he can have as much fun and fulfilment as I am having. I'll take care of the bacon-bringing-home business.

As the weeks tick by I am so excited and brimful of fantastic thoughts and ideas that I start sleeping less and less. When I do sleep I have strange half-wakeful dreams. The Norwegian wakes one early morning to find me tickling him under the chin. When he asks if I'm all right I say,

'I thought you were the baby. There is something about ... something about the woman having to check on the baby more'.

I have always been prone to this semi-sleep talk. One night when we first moved to Australia, I had had an early night. The Norwegian came in to give me a kiss goodnight but I was already half asleep. He knelt down to kiss me and I pushed him away.

'You are like an umbrella,' I snapped. He had a prickly three-day-old beard. Then, in my dazed state, realising that wasn't a very good reaction to a lovely bedtime kiss, I give him some constructive advice: 'Next time, kiss me with the soft of your bottom.'

One night I wake up four times to jump out of bed in a panic and race to The Boy's bassinet. I only have a vague memory of this, but on one occasion The Norwegian tells me, I jump out of bed and take the duvet with me waking him up. Another time The Norwegian wakes up with The Boy's cries only to find me sitting up in bed with my eyes closed. I say ponderously, 'I seem to be having some difficulty opening my eyes.'

* * *

My ups are becoming frantic: I have too many racing thoughts to manage. The scribbles in my beige notebook become less and less easy to understand. I scrawl diagrams on the cover with arrows linking different words and spend hours surfing the net, like people used to do in the '90s. Facebook becomes my site of choice as I try to track down long lost friends.

Later, one of my friends back in the UK, who had a baby a month before me, but was having a more normal experience of how hard it is having a young baby, said she couldn't quite understand how 'perky' I was in my Facebook updates. One of my updates said, 'Things I didn't expect about being a mum—more time to write, not less.' I didn't add that this was because my sleep hours were dwindling from five hours, to four, then to three.

A few weeks after the birth I got seriously constipated and duly started taking the supplement again. But this time the supplement wasn't working and, after a few days of the terrible feeling of things backing up virtually to my stomach, I finally managed to push out an enormous poo the girth and length of a Coke can.

As I was straining away, with The Doctor's voice ringing in my ears DONT GET CONSTIPATED and The Boy shouting away in the sitting room, the poo got stuck. It just wouldn't move. The rhythmical contracting and expanding of my bowel, known as peristalsis, had pretty much stopped half way. No matter how much I strained it wouldn't move and it was really hurting.

Eventually it came out and as I wiped myself, the tissue came away with blood so I booked a doctor's appointment for the next day.

Two words I never wanted to hear in the same sentence from my GP are anal and fissure. She told me that the supplement was bulking up my poo and, essentially, I'd just been making the poo bigger but not any softer. She prescribed me a stool softener rather than a bulking agent and a cream to help the fissure. Never again I promised my aching guts and compromised bottom. I discovered too late that there are two types of constipation needing different treatment.

* * *

I pump for a week after I leave the hospital and my nipples recover enough to start breastfeeding again. I'm a bit addicted to the *ammetåke* feeling from the breast pump and am happy to discover that, after the first toe-curling painful seconds, the same chilled-out, bliss feelings settle over me when I'm breastfeeding. I love the sight of my dark-haired boy snuggling at my breast, drinking his fill.

But, as it is still painful, I go to see one of the staff at the Early Childhood Health Care Clinic and get her to watch my latch. She gives me the thumbs up, but is worried I might have thrush on my nipples. She thinks this might be why they were hurting. Thrush is caused by fungus that occurs naturally in the body. It's usually kept under control by 'friendly' bacteria, but can occur in the baby's mouth and then be passed onto the mum's nipples while breastfeeding.

I also show her my less than gentle method for getting him off the breast and she says, 'Whatever works for you, darl.'

'I'm sort of getting used to the pain,' I say. But, seeing how easy other mothers are finding breastfeeding, I realise something is still not going well for us.

'It really shouldn't hurt that much,' she says.

The pain gets worse and worse and in Week Five I go back to expressing. You need to keep stimulating the breast to make sure your milk supply doesn't dry up. I am up twice a night to express then feed and, despite The Norwegian loyally getting up to help, it all adds to my sleeplessness. And, of course, once I was up I just have to check Facebook, as it's the middle of the day in the UK. It makes perfect sense to me.

People ask me how the baby is sleeping and I say, 'Fine', because he is a brilliant sleeper. But no one asks me how *I* am sleeping. And therein lies the rub.

The psychosis

'Dr Martin Luther King said, "I have a dream" and then he woke up.'

My Diary Entry

Chapter Nine

It all starts with Renée Zellweger. Before The Boy's arrival I chat to one of our neighbours, a lovely lady in her sixties with a silver bob and bright eyes. She's from England and swims in the sea every day no matter what the weather. As we chat, both folding our respective washing from the line, she tells me her daughter—whose child is due around the same time as ours—is coming over from LA to stay with her.

'How wonderful,' I'd say.

'She's an actor.'

'Really cool.'

This fact lodges itself deep in my brain.

It is Monday of Week Six and as we are leaving the apartment I see a woman clutching a very small baby. *Ah*, I think, *that must be the daughter. Her face looks very familiar.*

That morning we have the six-week check with The Obstetrician. This, as the name suggests, is a health check for mother and baby around the six-week mark. The Norwegian is going in to work late so he can come with me. While waiting in the reception I flick through a copy of *Grazia* and see a photo of a woman clutching a small baby. It looks exactly like my neighbour's daughter. I check the name by the picture. Renée Zellweger.

It isn't a very flattering shot; she's wearing thick-rimmed glasses and her already small eyes are squinted into raisins in her round pale face. It is also quite blurry like it was shot from a distance and the photo editor had magnified it many times.

'Oh, my God,' I say to The Norwegian. 'I think Renée Zellweger is in our building. She's our neighbour's daughter.'

'I don't think so, Jen,' says The Norwegian. 'Are you feeling OK?'

'Yes, sure—I'm just so happy.'

* * *

I carry on flicking through the magazine and hit on another photo which stops me in my tracks.

'Look—it's one of your old college friends,' I wave the magazine at The Norwegian. It is a photo of the new mystery man in Sandra Bullock's life. He looks exactly like a crazy party-hound The Norwegian used to know.

'No, it isn't.'

'Yes it is.'

'It isn't, Jen. That isn't him.'

'But it looks exactly like him—and he knows famous people doesn't he.'

'He does, yes. But that's not him.' He turns back to his iPhone to check his work emails.

I know it's him. The Norwegian just isn't looking properly. He works too hard. I turn the page and see a photo of Halle Berry—wait, that looks just like my old school friend. I stare at the photo. I haven't seen her in a while and maybe she's secretly living a double life in Tufnell Park, when she's not in LA. Then I see a picture of Lindsay Lohan and it is our friend Clare, married to The Norwegian's old friend from university, Peter.

The magazine seems to glow. I turn the next page as if I'm in the British Library handling Shakespeare's First Folio with white-gloved hands. How do I know all these famous people? This seems so odd. Then a thought occurs to me. Maybe I'm famous too.

I look around the waiting room and feel a great upwelling of happiness. I am beaming. I catch the eye of a mother and child opposite. She gives me a brief smile then looks away embarrassed. I notice one of the receptionists looking at me then quickly looking away.

Why is everyone acting so weirdly towards me? I wonder. I turn another page of the magazine and see a picture of Cameron Diaz. And she looks exactly like me.

Oh, my God, I'm Cameron Diaz. I look at The Norwegian and he smiles back at me. In the picture she is wearing the blue shirt and cut-off shorts that I wear all the time. *I must have come to Australia, like Renée, to get away from the paparazzi while we have our baby.*

I look at The Norwegian again and think, *The lucky bastard, he gets to have sex with Cameron Diaz/Me.*

I am tallish, and was slim before the baby came. I like surfing. I have blonde hair and I love dancing. These things prove I must be Diaz. My addled brain conveniently ignoring the things we don't have in common, like me not being a world-famous movie star who once went out with

Justin Timberlake.

You may think this doesn't make sense; I must know I'm not Cameron Diaz? But I don't and here's why. I think I'm Cameron Diaz, which is quite a mad thing to think, so I'm either mad or I *am* Cameron Diaz. I know I'm not mad; I survived Day Six. Therefore I must be the Cameron Diaz. You see? It is like a very simple mathematical equation.

'The doctor is ready for you now,' says the receptionist and I carefully put the magazine down and look at The Norwegian. I am blazing with happiness and a bit wobbly on my feet, as you might expect after discovering I'm a world-famous actress who has secretly moved to Australia to have a baby with her 'civilian' husband.

'How are you doing, Jen?' asks the doctor.

I smile a knowing smile at him. *So we are all just going to go along with my alias. That's fine by me.*

'Well my scar is still weeping a bit and sore in parts, but other than that I'm fine. I'm really happy actually.'

He smiles at me and The Norwegian.

'Let me take a look.'

I hop up onto the couch, lift my dress and roll down the top of my knickers.

'How is the little one?' he asks as he bends over my nether regions.

'He is a little angel—really the perfect baby.' The Boy gurgles in the buggy.

The Obstetrician looks at me and raises his eyebrows.

'Good. Then let's have a look here.' He pauses and frowns bending further over me to get a closer look. 'I think I know why your scar isn't healing properly.

'They've left part of the stitch in.'

'Oh.'

'I'm really sorry about this, Jen. I'll be having stern words with the hospital.'

'That's OK, everyone makes mistakes sometimes.'

'You'll need to take a course of antibiotics.'

'No problems.'

He reaches for some metal pincers and sets about pulling out what looks like a very manky piece of blue string. It breaks open two of the scabs which start to bleed again. He presses a pad of white cotton wool dressing to the wound.

'There, that should do it, Jen.'

He helps me to my feet and I rearrange my dress. I laugh and give him a wink. Should I just say it—we are safe here in his little office, no one is going to know if I just come out with it.

'I can't thank you enough for everything you've done. I'm so happy.' My famous megawatt smile almost blinds him. I bet it is pretty unnerving having such a famous patient.

We are clustered at the door of his office in an awkward bundle. He reaches his hand out, but I go for his cheek instead and he laughs. I imagine him telling his wife, *Cameron Diaz kissed me today*, and both laughing over it.

'You do seem very happy,' he says as he shakes The Norwegian's hand.

As we head down in the lift I give The Norwegian a massive hug. I can see us reflected in the polished metal of the lift wall and I stare in disbelief. I don't see Cameron Diaz's face staring back at me. It is just plain old Jen.

'I'm not Cameron Diaz, am I?' I ask.

The Norwegian pulls out of the hug and looks me hard in the face.

'Are you sure you're OK?'

'Yeah.' I laugh.

He frowns at me and I smile back at him.

'What do you mean then?'

'Oh nothing,' I say. 'Just a thought.'

*　*　*

Because what are delusions really but just thoughts from an over-active brain. The way I've always understood my sister's illness is that she had too much dopamine in her brain. Dopamine is one of a few neurotransmitters that help electrical impulses leap across the gap between brain cells. Having too much means that your brain makes too many leaps, and you start believing—as my sister did—that you can fly, communicate telepathically, or hear what the neighbours are really saying about you behind your back. Your brain literally jumps to conclusions.

Of course, the reality of schizophrenia is much more complex than just an overabundance of dopamine. If that was as simple as that, then we would have cured it by now. Scientists are still puzzling out this complex and devastating illness.

I once asked my sister about the voices she hears when her brain is misfiring.

'If you know they aren't real, can't you just ignore them?' I asked.

'OK, let's do an experiment,' she said.

'OK.'

'Talk to me. Just say anything you like.'

'Um ... well, it is lovely to see—'

'You're SHIT!' she hissed into my ear.

'What?'

'Go on, just ignore it.'

'Oh.'

'Go on. Try again.'

I was silent for a second. Her face was intent. *She really wants me to understand this.* So I tried again.

'I'm having a great—'

She moved to stand behind me and whispered into my ear:

'I'm behind you.' Her voice was quiet, filled with menace. 'Don't turn around or I'll—'

'Stop. Stop please. I think I get it. Is it really that bad?'

'Yes. Sometimes worse.'

'That's horrible, Jo.' I looked at her and she smiled back at me. My heart grew cold.

'That's what it's like. They sound as real as your voice does to me now.'

'How do you cope with it?' I asked humbled and scared.

She smiled and shrugged, and we carried on with our walk.

Chapter Jen

The next day is Tuesday and mothers' group looms. The Norwegian also works from home on a Tuesday.

I am having one of my downs begging The Norwegian to drive me to mothers' group.

'I can't do it on my own. You just have no idea how hard it is for me to drive with a baby in the car.'

'Don't worry, Jen, I'll drive you. It's only up the road.'

'It may only be up the road to you but it isn't for me. I have no idea if I'll find parking. It's ... it's ...'

'I said I'll take you, Jen.'

'OK, OK,' I say trying to calm down. 'Thanks,' I mutter, looking around the room. The fear grabs me again.

'I mean, I've no idea what I am supposed to pack to take with me.'

'Just what we normally pack: nappies, bottles and—'

'Oh, it's all so easy for you, isn't it? I can't do it. I CAN'T. Please help me.' I dissolve into tears.

The Norwegian gets up from his desk and comes over and takes my hand.

'You don't have to go if you don't want to.'

'But I have to get used to leaving the flat with The Boy. Otherwise it'll be terrible.'

'What will?'

'Everything.'

He calmly helps me pack up the nappy bag and makes sure I have everything: my phone, my wallet and keys.

'See, you'll be OK.'

'I'm so sorry, babes, I don't know what's wrong with me today. I feel so wired and anxious.'

We drive the short distance to the Early Childhood Health Care Clinic where the mothers' group is being held. The Norwegian drops me off and I take a deep breath and walk into the room.

I smile as I see one of the friendly women in the mpther's group, and the anxiety starts to ebb. *I can do this. I can do this.* I sit down and the Early

Childhood Nurse, smiles her hello. The room fills up and The Nurse starts her talk on settling techniques.

The room is rapt, listening intently.

'What do we do if they just keep waking up?' someone asks.

I laugh.

'Well, you just have to keep trying,' she says.

I laugh again. The Nurse glances at me with a concerned expression.

'What do you do if you have the best baby in the world?' I say.

Now everyone laughs. I pick up The Boy and hold him up. Everyone is looking at me. I am controlling the room. I can make them laugh if I laugh.

The Nurse starts talking again and the hour goes by in a blur. As all the others file out I grab her. The day before I'd booked her to do the The Boy's six-week check.

We go into her office. It overlooks the car park and I can see The Norwegian pacing up and down on the phone. Her office has a large L-shaped desk piled with papers and a counter along one of the walls with scales and nappy-changing equipment.

'Pop him up here on the scales.' She watches the display and jots down notes in our 'Blue Book'. This is a folder given to each new mum to keep track of their baby's growth, development and any medical issues. In the UK mums are issued with a 'Red Book'.

'He is a good weight,' she says as The Boy wiggles and squirms.

'Yes, he is a healthy, thriving boy.'

'Thank you, thank you,' I say relieved.

I go to leave and she puts her hand on my arm.

'And how are you?'

'I'm really good; not sleeping much but that is par for the course, isn't it?'

'Yes, it is I'm afraid. Are you having difficulty settling him?'

'No, he sleeps really well. It's me having trouble getting to sleep.'

'Really. Why?'

'I'm too excited, I guess. I love being a mum so much. I love it, love it, love it.'

She is silent.

I go to pick up The Boy and wave at The Norwegian through the window.

'Wait for a minute,' she says. 'Is that your partner?'

'Yes. He is half Norwegian. We got married last year. It was wonderful, really such a wonderful day.' My words are coming tumbling out over one another. I wave at him to come in.

After a few moments he knocks lightly on the door and comes into the room.

'All is well with The Boy,' I tell him.

'Good,'

'I have a book I want to recommend to you,' she says riffling through the papers on her desk.

'We should get going,' I say.

'Just one more minute,' she says. 'Where did you work before bubs?'

'At the Cerebral Palsy Alliance,' I say. 'They are such a great organisation. Have you heard of them?'

'Yes, they are marvellous.'

The Nurse is starting to get on my nerves. She won't stop asking me questions. I just want to leave.

'I'm going to wait in the car,' I say hoping this will hurry things up. I take The Boy with me and secure him into the car seat.

The Norwegian is taking ages. I can see them chatting through the window. I make a grimace when The Nurse is looking down at something on her desk.

'Come on,' I mouth.

What I didn't know was that The Nurse was stalling while she found the number of the Extended Hours Team—previously known as the Mental Health Crisis Team. There's a good name change, if ever I heard one.

She had started getting alarmed during the mothers' group.

'Is she always like this?' she asks The Norwegian.

'No, she's very much not like this. She's not getting much sleep.'

'I think something more serious is happening and I'd like you to ring the Extended Hours Team.' She hands over a yellow Post-it note with a number scrawled on it.

When we get back to our apartment, The Norwegian suggests I have a nap while he looks after The Boy. Gratefully I plunge into bed and fall into a fitful sleep.

An hour and a half later he comes to wake me up. Sitting on the edge of the bed he says,

'Jen, some people are coming around. We are all very worried about you and think you might need some help.'

'People. What do you mean?' My heart leaps. Fear grips me.

'They are from the Extended Hours Team.'

Even though they have changed the name, I still know what it means.

'No. No. No!' I inch back in the bed away from his calming hands.

'It's going to be all right, Jen.'

'No, it isn't. I'm going mad, aren't I? They are going to section me? Aren't they?'

'I won't let that happen.'

'You won't be able to do anything about it. This is really it, isn't it? I'm going mad.' I start to cry desperate tears and try to get out of bed.

'Jen, everything is going to be fine. They are here to help. I've explained at great length about your sister and your fear of going mad.'

He holds me tight and the tears spill and spill.

We hear a knock on the door.

'I'm going to get that, OK?'

He leaves the room and I sit in bed with the madness harrying me like a terrier, nipping and pulling. I grip the duvet tight and take a deep breath. I think about the help button in the hospital. Now my time really has come.

Chapter Eleven

I come out of the bedroom into the sitting room. There are two strange people—one sitting on our brown leather rocking chair and the other on the brown textured Ottoman.

They both smile at me.

'Hi, Jen, I'm from the Extended Hours Team,' says one. He is a stocky man with a barrel-like chest and a brown smiling face. He has a black briefcase like my mother used to have back in the 80s.

'I'm Claudette,' says the other. She is English with dark straight hair and a flick of eyeliner at the corner of each eye.

These two people sit in my home and look at me. I start crying and The Norwegian comes over to me.

'It's all right Jen, they are just here to help.'

'That's right. Can you tell us what's been going on?'

I sit still for a moment on the sofa next to The Norwegian.

'I think I'm losing my mind,' I say.

I tell them about my fear of going mad like my sister and that we are approaching the 15th March—the anniversary of her first breakdown.

'That sounds very tough, Jen. But what you are going through is nothing like schizophrenia.'

'Really? Are you sure?'

'Yes, absolutely.'

'What is it then?'

'We think it is caused by extreme sleeplessness.'

'OK, that makes sense.'

'We will give you some medication to help you sleep and recommend you give up breastfeeding so you can get good, long stretches of sleep. Your husband can give your son a bottle.'

'But I don't want to give up breastfeeding.'

They ask me some questions about how I'm feeling within myself, towards The Boy.

'I know this is hard to hear but have you had any thoughts of harming yourself?'

'No.'

'Or harming anyone else? Your son?'

'God, no.'

They are calm, gentle and kind. They aren't going to make me do anything I don't want to do, I realise. I talk about thinking I was Cameron Diaz and they laugh along with me.

'It is a very strange feeling,' I say.

'You probably should stop reading those gossip mags,' says Claudette.

Eventually after what feels like hours of talking back and forth they prescribe temazepam, a sedative used to treat insomnia.

'We recommend that you stop breastfeeding while you catch up on sleep, and while taking these drugs,' says Claudette.

'So I should just express milk until I stop taking the medication and can go back to breastfeeding?'

'We don't know how long it will take.'

'I don't want to stop breastfeeding,' I say again. 'I need to carry on.'

'Jen, it is more important your son has a well mother than breastmilk.'

Even though I don't think there is anything wrong with bottle-feeding, I am consumed with sadness at the idea I have to forgo breastfeeding.

They also want me to stop taking the amitriptyline as it is a mood elevator and my mood is already quite elevated. They say they will keep monitoring me.

'You should be fine once you've caught up on sleep.' Claudette flips open the black briefcase and hands over one pill. I hold it in the palm of my hand. One small tablet that I must take. I look up at Claudette again and he smiles reassuringly back at me.

'My sister used to be very resistant about taking her meds,' I say gulping the pill. They both smile at me.

'What you have is nothing like your sister's illness, you have to remember that.' says Claudette.

It feels like they will never leave. There is silence and they all look at me.

'Well thanks for coming over,' I say. It is all I can think of. The Norwegian gives me a wonky look.

As we finally shut the door behind them The Norwegian pulls me into a big hug.

'See, that was OK.'

'I thought they'd never go.'

'You are going to be OK, do you believe that now?'

I shrug.

What I don't know is that after their visit they ring The Norwegian and tell him I could be a risk to The Boy and to myself. They tell him not to leave me on my own with The Boy, or on my own, full stop.

Over the next week we are visited by two people, twice a day. The Norwegian has to take the week off work. Twice a day we sit on the sofa and everyone looks at me as I tell them what I am going through. They ask questions and I answer to the best of my ability.

During each visit time drags. Despite their kindness and professional concern I feel their scrutiny like ants on my skin. I am convinced that they won't go unless The Norwegian or I actually ask them to. I feel that I can't ask them, as they might start wondering what I have to hide, so we work out a system. When I go to the bathroom, The Norwegian knows this is my signal for him to wrap up the conversation.

At first, they say what I am experiencing is caused by sensitivity to the incredible hormone soup racing around my body, as well as a severe lack of sleep. And for the first two days things seem to calm down once I get a couple of decent nights' sleep. 'You must protect your sleep,' they tell me. 'That is really important.'

But then, despite the meds and the restorative sleep, by the end of the week things start getting worse again, and they start talking about postpartum psychosis (PPP). This term covers a collection of mental illnesses that occur once or twice in every thousand births. Robin Barker says in *Baby Love*, 'With prompt recognition and correct treatment, postnatal psychosis has an excellent prognosis with full recovery in a few months.'

They try me on a new drug, an anti-psychotic called olanzapine. They prescribe it for my mania and delusions. It is the same drug my sister used to take when she was first ill. It was developed as a treatment for schizophrenia and bipolar disorder, but it can also be used as a mood stabiliser and for the general treatment of psychosis.

My fear of going mad like my sister is not helped by taking the same drug she used to take. It is a big deal. A very big deal. I feel frightened and hopeless even though I know I need to take the medication to get better.

As I am no longer breastfeeding, in theory I should get a full night's sleep with The Norwegian feeding The Boy formula. But I am still pumping as I can't give up the idea of breastfeeding. I wake up when The Norwegian creeps back into bed. He tells me later he would sit in the bedroom listening to me move around the flat, bone tired but fearful of what I might do. He would get up and sometimes find me in The Boy's room with the lights blazing staring down at our little son. Sometimes I would pick him up, usually just after The Norwegian had spent hours trying to settle him. Once I just stood in front of the fridge until The Norwegian gently lead me back to bed. Another time I shut The Boy's bedroom door in The Norwegian's face and wouldn't let him in.

Other nights I would stay up watching episodes of *Thirty Rock* over and over again. I became convinced that because my brain was working at such a high level now, I was somehow seeing each individual frame of film. I could even 'see' so fast that I could see frames of film that the editor hadn't cut quite enough. I'd replay the same episode over and over, 'seeing' more and more of these 'out-takes'. I thought I saw unscripted interaction between Tina Fey and the other actors that was funnier than the rest, which is already pretty effing hilarious. I thought that Kenneth was one of my uni friends and that I went to school with Dot Com.

I also watched YouTube videos of De La Soul songs over and over. I became convinced that my first boyfriend at school was Plug One and that all De La Soul songs were messages to me from him. I was particularly hooked on 'Three is a magic number' as I thought this was very significant. I was convinced that three really was the magic number because of what had happened to me at the maternity hospital. I thought that it had happened on the third day of The Boy's life rather than the sixth. But, when I checked my diary and found out that it was in fact Day Six, it didn't phase me: I just thought, well, six is just twice three so it is doubly the magic number.

I know now that when you are having delusions you will twist all things around to make your delusion right. The conviction the delusion is real is so strong that reality warps around it like light around a black hole. It has made me much more understanding of my sister when she clings to, what I think are delusions, but she thinks are real.

Not all my delusions and manic thoughts were unpleasant; in fact, some of the time I felt euphoric. However, this period was by far the hardest time for The Norwegian, being so worried in case the psychiatric nurses were right and I was a danger to The Boy or myself. Some women with postpartum psychosis hear voices telling them to hurt their child or themselves. I'm lucky, in the midst of such overarching bad luck, that this didn't happen to me.

Chapter Twelve

It is the middle of the night. The Norwegian is feeding The Boy as I'm pumping. I still can't give up the hope that I'll be able to go back to breastfeeding when all this is over.

I slip back into bed with The Norwegian. We both lie there awake. He is waiting for me to fall asleep, but the exhaustion of the last few days catches up with him and he slips under. I, as tired as I am, lie awake listening to his breathing.

The walls and ceiling are moving, bending. I breathe in and the walls bend towards me, breathe out and they shimmer back into place. I know I'm not mad but, if I'm sane, then the walls really are moving. What if the walls are appearing to move for some other unknown reason? But what could it be? I breathe in and the room contracts again, breathe out and it expands.

I silently get up and close the door as The Norwegian rolls over in his sleep. I go and check on The Boy. He is flat on his back, sparked out. I watch him. His breath rasps quietly like a velvet cricket. The room blurs and shimmers in the dark.

I go into the bathroom and splash my face with water. It is 2.30 am. I hear a thump against the bathroom door and I spin around. Nothing. I lean over the sink. Get a grip, Jen; get a grip.

The pink and blue square tiles on the floor start jumping and moving. Shapes fall like Tetris. I grip the edge of the sink and the room swirls around me. I slowly lift my face to the mirror and see someone else's face. She looks like me but has a smaller button nose and grey eyes where my blue ones should be. There is a stripe of red down the side of her face. It is throbbing. I lift my hand, and she lifts hers, too, as we both feel the tenderness around the red raised bump.

I turn around and look at the white painted bathroom door. It is blurring and changing colour as I hear another thump. The door is now scrubbed pine.

I start to pant and lean on the sink. It is 1962. He is just outside. I know that. The handle turns slowly.

'Annie,' he calls in a rough whisper.

'Annie, no need to hide. I'll be gentle with you.'

The handle turns again and he rattles the door.

'Undo the lock Annie. Come on girl. We both know this is going to happen. I've seen the way you look at me.'

* * *

They'd both been smashed drunk when they came in a few hours earlier; my husband Tom and his friend Jack. Friday meant one thing for them, pay day and the pub. I'd tried to serve them up the stew I'd made but they both laughed and slapped the table.

'Eating is cheating,' said Jack.

'We're thirsty not hungry,' Tom laughed. He had opened up a bottle of whisky and placed it on the table between the plates of rapidly cooling stew. They'd drunk and drunk, their talk getting louder and louder. It was all about the boss they called Captain and all the ways he was a failure: nitpicking, penny-pinching, no-good weakling.

I left them to it and got started on the washing up. I could hear their raucous voices getting louder and louder as I rinsed the plates in the soapy water. Then I noticed it had fallen quiet and I realised, with a jolt, that Jack was standing leaning in the kitchen doorway.

'You know you are a fine looking woman, Annie,' he'd said.

'Jack, that's the drink—' I started when he lunged at me catching me with his open hand around the side of my face. But in his drunkenness he misjudged the distance and crashed into the side of the sink. In a flash I had twisted away from him and run to the bathroom, slamming the door and turning the key just as he came stumbling after me.

'You bitch, let me in,' he says, and starts banging the door in earnest. The lock is holding, for now.

And where was Tom in all this? Probably passed out drunk in his chair.

Jack bangs again and the wood around the lock starts to splinter.

'Tom!' I scream. 'Tom, where are you?'

'Tom!'

'TOM!'

With each cry Jack attacks the door with renewed vigour, kicking at the lock. The wood splinters further and further with each kick.

'I'm almost in,' says Jack in between heavy breaths.

Then I hear an almighty roar: 'JACK'.

And then a heavy thud and slide.

'Get out—get out!' Tom yells.

'She led me on Tom, you know what she's like.'

'GET. OUT. NOW!'

I hear the front door open and bang shut.

'Annie, it's me. You're OK now.'

'Am I?' I shout. 'Where were you? How could you bring this into our home?'

'He's gone now Annie. It is safe to come out.'

I lean my head against the door.

'Is he gone?' I reach down for the lock. The key has gone and in its place a simple slide lock. I crease my brows.

'Tom?' I call to silence.

The door is changing again, back to the thick white paint; the pine has gone. I slide open the lock and the kitchen—familiar, dark and empty—is all that is waiting for me. I touch my face and the swelling has disappeared. I am back in the now.

I go and sit on the rocking chair staring out of the windows into the dark night. My hands rest loosely together in my lap. Our apartment is high up over the Manly to Spit Bridge scenic walk, and in the day we have views over to The Heads and across to Forty Baskets beach. The Heads are two rocky headlands, one north, one south, that flank the entrance to Sydney Harbour. Now, though, all is dark, apart from the green light on a marker buoy, which flashes on; flashes off.

I am calm again. Whatever is coming I can deal with. I take a deep breath and release it in a big sigh. I rock backwards and forwards in the rocking chair.

The room around me fades away. The windows and walls softly melt and turn into dark leaves and branches. Just like Max's bedroom in *Where the Wild Things Are*.

I am up high in the branches of a paper-bark tree. I reach out and touch the flaky bark with my outstretched hand. My skin is dark black. I am an Aboriginal woman. It is 1788.

The dark night lightens. The stars and moon fade and a golden twilight illuminates the undersides of the clouds.

I can see the green-cloaked headland of North Heads fronted by the yellow sand of Spring Cove. The buildings around the beach that make up the Quarantine Station are gone. The gap of open ocean is framed on the other side by the craggy cliffs of South Head. The buildings on South Head are also gone. All around me is pristine bush with waving branches and twinkling water.

This is the entrance to our territory. The territory of Guringai people, my people. The sky lightens more until it is the sparkling light of late morning. I see a great canoe coming in through the heads. It has thick straight poles, the height of trees, decorated by large bright flashes of white cloths. The canoe seems to move without paddles, blown by the winds of the sea. I have never seen anything like it.

'It is so big,' I say to Banjora who is in the tree next to me.

'Yes,' he says. 'The biggest I've ever seen.'

The wind rustles the silver and green leaves bringing the breath of the ocean, scented with eucalyptus.

'We must tell the Elders about this,' he says as we climb backwards down the tree. He gives me a light kiss and we set off at a fast-paced run.

The Elders quickly gather two groups to run in either direction along the waterline to see where this strange canoe is going to land. I go with the first group and Banjora goes with the second. I am running fast along the path that skirts the water's edge. I feel the earth slapping against my feet as we race along. We get to a narrow sandy beach, on the north side of the water. It is a perfect landing spot; we wait out of sight in the bush.

The canoe looks even larger now, so big, so big. It is big enough to have a smaller, rounder canoe attached to it. We can see men, white men, scrambling all over the canoe. Some are climbing down into one small canoe. They pull it along towards the beach with long straight paddles. The men are wearing cloth coverings all over their bodies and the sound of their unfamiliar calls carries over the water.

As they pull the canoe up onto the sand we step out of the bush. They freeze and then cluster closer together in a tight knot. I can hear the gibberish that is their language as they talk to one another.

'What do you want here?' asks Killara, the eldest in our group.

They shout and laugh. Some of the men point at me and the other women. One of them moves his hands to his chest, hands curving. A gust of wind blows their smell over to us: grim sweat and rotten fish. Three of them are holding blunt metal staffs that appear to be their weapons. We have our spears.

One of them steps forward with his hand raised. His face is burnt deep red and his eyes are like two fragments of the sky. He has a hat made of stiff, black material and a dark blue cloak over his body. He makes the motion of a cup tipping into his mouth.

'Waa-ter, waa-ter,' he says.

The other men are collecting together in a tight knot behind him with their metal staffs pointing out towards us. One of the men points at me again and says something that makes all the other men laugh. The leader quiets them with a harsh word.

'You are not welcome here,' says Killara stepping forward.

One of the metal staffs explodes with a flash and Killara is knocked off his feet, a great gaping hole in his stomach. He screams in pain. Dragging him back we retreat into the trees but the men come running after us. One of them grabs my arm pulling me towards the small canoe.

A great spear flashes past me into the man's side. I turn and see Banjora as he pulls the spear out of the fallen man's body. He grabs my hand and pulls me away down the track. There are two more thunderclaps from the white men's metal staffs. We run swiftly back along the path.

As I run I realise I am still. I can feel the earth, leaves and twigs beneath my feet and my back resting on the rocking chair. My chest is heaving from running and it is calm and measured at the same time. In softly and out relaxed. The fright and the pain fade away.

I look around and I'm back in the room. *I am regressing through my past lives.* So the Buddhists are right, we do come back to this planet over and over again until we learn what we need to learn. I sense I'm so close to nirvana, but I don't want to go. I feel a great weight of sadness thinking if I disappeared into nirvana I'd never see The Boy or The Norwegian again. Then I realise my attachment to the two men in my life means I will stay firmly on the earth, and I breathe a sigh of relief.

The room starts to blur and shimmer again. I can feel myself spiralling back though time; *The Big Bang* credits in reverse. Back, back, back I go. Time whirling about me. Back before there were roads, before we built the pyramids, before Christ was born, back, back, back.

I'm still surrounded by leaves and branches. The morning sun lights patches on the ground. I look down and stroke my forearm. I am covered in dark soft fur, with pink hairless palms. My arms are incredibly strong. I lift my hands to my face and feel the fur on my cheeks and forehead. I look to my left and oo oo my lips into a monkey pout. I see another like me standing next to me. We are in a clearing in a dense forest.

I am Eve the first human and my mate standing next to me is my Adam. I hold out my hand and he takes it in his, stroking the back with his long fingers. He turns to me and says the first words ever spoken.

'I love you.'

'I love you,' I say back.

'Jen,' I hear. The trees and earth fade away and the night draws in around me again.

I'm back in the sitting room and The Norwegian is rubbing his eyes and coming out of the bedroom.

'What are you doing up?'

'Weird things are happening,' I say. He kneels before me holding my hands.

'What things?'

'I understand so much now,' I say.

'Come to bed.'

'I know why the caged bird sings.'

'Jen, please.'

Chapter Thirteen

It is Friday afternoon and The Norwegian and I are arguing again.

'Please, just look at this. It will explain everything.' I thrust my notebook at him. He looks down at the diagram.

'Well, do you get it now? Do you understand why all arguments are circular?'

He looks up at me sadly and says nothing.

'Well?'

'No, Jen, I don't but ...'

'I can't stand it any more. You must understand it. It is so clear. We've been over and over this. You must get it.'

'I'm sorry but it just doesn't make sense.'

'It is so obvious. All arguments are circular because they are. That proves it.'

He says nothing.

'It is saying that one person always has to give in. Even this argument is circular. I should give in because then you'll see. But I can't give in because it is so important that you understand.'

'Jen, I ...' he trails off.

There is a silence and I look at him hard, thinking, say it. Over the last few days I'd been trying to get him to say a certain phrase to reassure me.

'I'm strong, you are strong and you are not going mad.' I make him say this to me over and over.

'Say it'

'I am strong, you are strong and you are not going mad.'

'Say it like you mean it.'

'I do mean it.'

'SAY IT!'

'I *am* strong, you are strong and you are not going mad.'

'Say it like you mean it, say it like you mean it, sayitlikeyoumeanit, sayitlikeyoumeanit. SAY IT!

'I am strong you are strong and you are NOT going mad.'

'That's it. I've had enough. You can't even say the one thing I need to hear with conviction,' I shout.

I open the front door and step out onto the landing outside our apartment. We are five stories up. I flip my leg over the handrail.

'You need to understand how desperate I am. I *need* you to understand me.'

Finally, finally I push The Norwegian too far, the most patient and loving man I have ever met has reached his limit. He grabs me and pulls me away from the edge.

'Don't do that,' he shouts pulling me inside the apartment.

'I wasn't going to jump I just needed you to understand.'

'Never do that again.'

I don't remember this. The Norwegian only told me when I was much better and able to deal with the feeling of horror at what I'd put him through. He decided not to tell any of the health professionals that I'd done this. He says it wasn't like I was really going to jump but that I was just so desperate for him to understand me. He felt, if he told them, I'd be under even more scrutiny and we were only just coping with two visits a day.

In desperation The Norwegian calls my oldest friend in Australia, Lautaro. We were in the same class in school and originally made friends because of a mutual love of Stephen King books. He is like the brother I never had.

The Norwegian, close to tears explains what has been happening and that he is at the end of his endurance. I am in the other room and hear nothing of the conversation.

'We keep on arguing; she won't listen to me and is being more and more aggressive.'

'What can I do to help? Anything at all, just ask.'

'Could you call her and have a chat?'

'Sure and I'll see if I can come and say hello next week.'

Later that day my phone rings. It is Lautaro. I sit in the rocking chair looking out at the sea and sunshine outside. I pour out all my strange thoughts; my first boyfriend, is Plug One from De La Soul; how it all revolves around pelicans; and how I'm going to write a bestseller and so is he.

'Whose will be best?' he asks, and I laugh.

'Mine. But yours will be pretty good too. Like *The Beach* by Alex Garland only funnier.'

He listens to me with the occasional, *yes I see*. And *so I hear you saying*

... he just lets me go on and on emptying my mind of crazy thoughts and improbable images.

'Jen, if you need anything, you know you just need to ask.'

'It is so great to just talk to you. I knew you'd understand.'

'I'll pop by next week, then.' he says.

'See you then.'

The next day I am peaceful again in the morning and I decide to go for a walk.

'Are you sure you're OK?' The Norwegian asks.

'Yes. I'm feeling much calmer today.'

We hug and I close the door of our apartment behind me.

It is a crisp and beautiful morning and, as I walk along the Manly scenic walkway to North Harbour Reserve, I feel the stress and strain ebb away. As I walk along I realise I am surrounded by the humming and buzzing of the trees and plants. I look up above me and see branches leaning over the walkway, swaying in the breeze.

On one tree I see a curled, dried leaf the size of my hand. It is wedged in the crook of a branch. It is shaped like a boat washed up against the tree by the tide and the wind. It is filled with rainwater. I stop to marvel. *This is an important Aboriginal artefact.* It has probably been resting in the crook of that tree for hundreds of years, filling with rain at every shower and slowly draining away in the hot bright days of years gone by.

Then it hits me. This walkway is probably a sacred Songline for the Aboriginal people who lived around here before white Europeans arrived. Songlines are also known as Dreaming tracks by some Aboriginal communities. They mark the routes followed by creator-beings during the Dreaming, when the earth was first made. They are sung from generation to generation, and are like aural maps used to navigate by landmarks, hills, waterholes and deserts.

This was the path that my ancestor ran down when she saw Captain Cook's boat. I saw it all, so it must be true.

The path undulates under my feet as I take step after magical step. I am surrounded by beauty, nature at her best, with the thick undergrowth a glossy dark green. I pass a fragrant jasmine bush and the smell transports me back to summer holidays in Cyprus with my family when the parents let us teenagers camp out at Goat Beach.

As I move forward I spy a small nail on the edge of the path. This nail is from the early convict days I think. It is an important artefact and I must collect it and keep it safe. I pick it up and slip it into my pocket. Then I spot a piece of charcoal that is made of burnt bamboo. Another artefact. I can't believe that no one has noticed these important items on one of the busiest walkways in Sydney. By the time I get to the North Harbour Reserve I have half a dozen items in my pockets and hands.

As I go down the steps that lead onto the North Harbour Reserve a large pelican wheels overhead. She holds her wings steady and rides the thermals.

The reserve is a large expanse of grass with four great trees and a children's playground. It is bordered on three sides by trees, roads and houses, and on the fourth by an expanse of mud flats and shallow water. Standing on the grass in the middle of the reserve I put down my collection of artefacts. I let the breeze play over my outstretched arms and close my eyes.

I wish The Norwegian was with me. He would finally be able to understand. I almost race back to get him but then realise it is important for me to stay standing just here with the wind blowing through my body, cleansing me, making my mind clear and focused.

I sit down and a small dog comes running up to me and drops a ball at my feet. I pick up the ball and throw it back to the owner, but the dog returns to me dropping the ball again and looking up at me expectantly. I throw the ball again. And again. But each time the dog comes straight back. I point at the ground in front of my feet and the dog drops the ball and it rolls toward me. I realise that *I can control this dog with my mind.*

I look around at the four other dogs around the reserve. There are two labradoodles, one golden retriever and one cattle dog. I can control them all if I want to. I see the dogs all around me, weaving and running, fetching and returning, making a beautiful pattern over the grass that only I can see.

I am struck by a sudden idea. I work at the Cerebral Palsy Alliance and one of my roles is raising funds for prevention and cure research. We have a team of researchers at our Institute who really believe prevention and cure is possible in our lifetimes. One of these researchers is working on mapping the causal pathways of cerebral palsy. This is the special sequence of events that have to happen, in a certain order, for cerebral palsy to occur. One of the causal factors we are looking into is the impact of a bacterial or viral infection in the mother while the baby is in the womb.

I have a brainwave that perhaps the infection could come from gum disease. Many people have bleeding gums when they brush their teeth and don't think anything of it. So pregnant women would probably not think to mention it to doctors or anyone looking into the reasons why their child developed cerebral palsy. Maybe this is one of the causal factors and we didn't realise it because we had no data on it.

The wonderful thought occurs: *I'm going to cure cerebral palsy with dental floss.* I'll probably get a Nobel Prize for that one. Imagine all the emotional and physical pain that will be avoided once we know all women have to do is floss to get rid of gum disease while they are pregnant. I can't wait to ring work and tell them.

I've never felt such peace. I stand up and slowly start walking towards the stairs, back to our apartment, The Norwegian and The Boy. I know now, with this new calmness, I will be able to explain everything to The Norwegian.

As I walk back I notice something. Everyone I pass is looking at me. As I stare back at them, they look away. I see two joggers running towards me. Two tall and beautiful blondes, one touches her ear and says something into the hidden microphone. As they run towards me I smile and they look away. I know what's going on. They must be security laid on by Renée to protect her from paparazzi and stalkers. That must be why there is so much security around here.

I see a man lying on the grass by the side of the path with sunglasses and a baseball hat. I see an older but fit looking couple walking their dog. I see a man kayaking out on the water. All of them. All of them are security personnel.

The day before I'd seen a friend from my year at school on the grass in front of our apartment. He has large and beautiful eyes and dark smooth skin. We'd all had a crush on him back in those days. He was pretending to give personal training to a woman who was also part of his team. I stared at them until they both smiled up at me.

I'd been messaging him on Facebook. He must have thought it was so funny being in touch with me, pretending to be back in London, when he was actually in Australia. I could tell from the photos on Facebook that he is now running a personal security company for very high profile clients. But the amount of bodyguards around does seem a bit much for just one famous actress.

When I return I find The Norwegian watching a World Cup rugby match with The Boy gurgling on his mat. I tuck myself in next to him on the sofa after I've made both of us a cup of tea. He is intently watching the match so I think I'll explain things to him later.

I'm on Facebook that evening as The Norwegian baths, bottles and beds The Boy. I'm looking at Facebook again. One of my friend has posted a picture of Barack Obama shaking hands with someone. I stare at the picture and the other person starts to wobble and fade. I realise that, in the future, it's going to turn into me.

That is why there is so much security around. Barack Obama is coming to meet me. Renée has organised it. But why? For the life of me I can't work it out. I look over at The Norwegian. He is feeding The Boy his bottle sitting in the rocking chair. He has a faraway expression, gently rocking backwards and forwards murmuring to The Boy in Norwegian. I decide not to tell him, let it be a surprise for him.

We have arranged to Skype with my parents at seven so I load up Skype. My parents' faces fill the screen. I can't wait to tell them everything. They'll be so pleased.

The Norwegian holds The Boy up to the camera on the laptop and my parents coo and wave.

'Hello,' I say, as The Norwegian takes The Boy off to bed. Then I notice there are curtains behind them I don't recognise.

'Where are you?' I say.

'At the cottage,' says Mum.

'I don't recognise the curtains.'

'We usually Skype in the kitchen. We are in the sitting room this morning.'

'Where are you really?' I ask. Mum sets her lips into a straight line.

'We are at the cottage,' she repeats. 'Really, love.'

Then it hits me. They are in Australia! They are downstairs in my neighbour's flat. Renée had been talking to Lindsay Lohan and they thought it would be a lovely surprise if my parents were around to meet Obama too. After all, I am the person I am today because of my parents.

'Are you downstairs?' I ask.

'No,' says Dad his brow furrowed. 'We really are at the cottage.'

I guess they don't want to spoil the surprise so I go along with them.

A few weeks ago my sister had sent me a present. It was a 1956 edition of *The Sea Around Us* by Rachel Carson. She is best known for her seminal book, *Silent Spring*, credited with sparking the environmental movement.

'Hey, guess what,' I say, 'Jo sent me a really marvellous present.'

'Did she?'

'Yeah it is by a really famous author. I think it might be worth a lot of money. I've emailed Christies' rare book department and they are getting back to me with a valuation.'

'Jen!' says Mum.

'Don't you think Jo will be so pleased once I find out exactly how much it is worth. I think it is probably worth at least a million pounds.'

My parents are silent. The room darkens as the sun slips below Balgowlah Heights to the west.

''I'll go and get it,' I say going over to the bookcase and gently sliding the book out. I see another book next to it. *Lucky Jim* by Kingsley Amis. *Lucky Jim* I think. My Dad's called Jim. I stare at the cover picture. It has a line drawing of a man standing in front of a Cambridge college holding two books: *Toynbee* and *A Short History of Economic Theory*. It looks exactly like Dad.

This is so exciting. This means this book is worth a lot of money too. I wonder how Dad will like being famous once everyone finds out *Lucky Jim* is based on him.

'How are you?' my mum asks The Norwegian.

'OK, pretty tired.'

'Here it is,' I wave the Rachel Carson book in front of the camera. 'But I've just made another discovery. Dad, have you read the book *Lucky Jim*?'

'Yes. I studied it in school in fact.'

'I have a copy here and Dad I think it is based on you.'

They both laugh out loud.

'I'm serious. Look at the picture, it looks just like you.'

'No, Jen, that's not possible. I studied it at school, so it was published when I was a boy. It couldn't be based on me, I'm too young.'

'But it must be you.'

'It can't be, Jen.'

'Have you read it?' asks Mum.

'No, not yet.'

'Then how do you know it is based on Dad?'

'Why won't you believe me? Why won't you all just believe what I say for once? It is so exhausting.'

Mum and Dad glance at each other. Then my mum leans forward towards The Norwegian sitting next to me.

'You must call for help. Call for help now.'

Psychosis comes from the Greek words *psyche* for mind or soul and *-osis* for diseased or abnormal condition. People with psychosis often have delusional beliefs and hallucinations. Hearing voices is a very common type of hallucination, which I was, thankfully, spared. My sister was not so lucky.

There is a knock at the door. It is the Extended Hours Team. We invite them in and explain that we are Skyping with my parents.

'We thought it would alleviate some of the anxiety for Jen's parents if we Skyped all together, then they can ask you questions,' says The Norwegian.

They pull a bench up to the desk so we are sitting in a horseshoe shape around the laptop.

'How are you doing today, Jen?'

'I'm OK but I did have quite a weird experience earlier today.'

'What was that?'

'I went for a walk and everyone was looking at me, but looked away when I looked at them. They were all security personnel. For tomorrow.'

'What is happening tomorrow?'

'I'm sure you know. No need to pretend.'

'No, I'm afraid we don't.'

'Oh, and I found this book that my sister gave me and I think it is worth a lot of money.'

'Jen, what do you think is going to happen tomorrow?'

'We are going to meet Obama. Together we are going to use Facebook to catch all paedophiles.'

There is silence.

'Jen,' says my mum, 'lots of strange things are happening to you. But if you, and I mean both of you, want me to come out, I will.'

'I think we'll be OK,' I say. 'Once everyone finally understands what I am trying to explain I think everything will be great. You'll see.'

The staff from the Extended Hours Team sit and talk with my parents answering questions about what is happening to me. After a while, I ask for my medication.

'I want to take it in front of my parents so they can see.'

They flip open the black briefcase and take out two boxes. They pop four tablets out of their blister packs and hand them over to me. One olanzapine, one temazepam and two of an anticonvulsant called sodium valproate which is used to treat epilepsy as well as a mood stabiliser. They started me on the sodium valproate earlier in the week.

'Look,' I say to my parents, 'I'm being compliant.'

'Good,' laughs Mum. 'Well done,' says Dad.

'Jen, I can see you are being very well looked after,' says Mum.

'Yes everyone has been very kind. Though sometimes people stay too long,' I smile.

'That's our cue, I think.'

'Lovely to meet you,' says Mum. 'And thanks for looking after our daughter so well.'

After we've finished talking to Mum and Dad, and everyone has left, The Norwegian and I sit on the sofa tucking into another takeaway meal.

'It will be OK, you know that?' he says.

'With you by my side everything is possible,' I say.

Chapter Fourteen

Saturday dawns bright. I am starting to catch up with sleep and feel more rested.

'How are you today?' asks The Norwegian

'OK. I feel less tired, but I'm still having such strange thoughts.'

'Sorry to hear that.'

He has dark circles under his puffy eyes. I know that me catching up on my sleep means he is getting less. I feel a stab of guilt and tuck the feeling away with all the others of the last few weeks.

After our morning visit from the Extended Hours Team I make a cup of tea. The flat is peaceful and quiet, but then I hear a sound coming from The Boy's room. I find The Norwegian sitting on the day bed with his face in his hands. He is crying quietly.

'What's wrong?'

'They said ...' he falters.

I put my arms around him and rest my cheek against his.

'I'm so sorry, you must be exhausted.'

'It's not that. I mean, yes, I'm knackered. It's just, last week they said, they said that you might be a risk to The Boy.'

He dissolves into crying again and I hug him tight.

'I didn't know whether to tell you or not,' he says.

'I don't think I am.'

'No, not when you're like this, but when you are in a bad place you just ... we just ... I don't know how much more I can take.'

We sit in silence holding tight to one another. The Norwegian takes a deep breath and wipes the tears from his eyes.

'It is just so hard,' he says, and my heart turns to lead in my chest.

'This is all my fault.'

'No. It isn't anyone's fault; it's just so hard. But I tell you what, let's make the most of you feeling OK and go and get a coffee. I can start talking really fast.'

The Norwegian is a coffee lover. I love that he loves coffee because when he has one he starts talking nineteen to the dozen about all and everything.

So we load up the buggy and brave the steepness of Woods Parade. At the top of the hill is the little row of shops that makes up Fairlight CBD. There is a butcher, a café, pharmacist, bottle shop, grocer, dry cleaner and a little bakery. The butcher's has a café attached with tables out on the pavement. We sit down at the one free table. The other tables throng with families with golden-haired children. They squeal and play around us with the sun glinting off their shining heads. I smile at The Norwegian. He smiles back and then starts playing with The Boy. Where's Papa? Here's Papa!

A cloud passes over the sun and the shining heads dim to shade. A cooler breeze puffs along the row of shops. A man with long dark hair pulled back into a stringy ponytail is walking backwards and forwards along the pavement. He is sauntering slowly, rolling each foot down, with his hands clasped behind his back. As he walks he looks at each child. His face is blank.

A chill creeps up from my stomach. Something is very wrong with this man.

'Look at him.' I say.

'Who?'

'That man. What is he doing?'

'He does look a bit suss,' The Norwegian laughs.

'He is scoping out those children. We have to warn them.'

'No, I think he works here, look he's wearing an apron.'

'That's probably what he wants people to think.'

I stand up and start towards the mother on the next table. The Norwegian grabs my hand.

'No, Jen.'

'But we have to.'

'No, please. Look, he has stopped now.'

The man has walked into the butcher's café and is leaning against the edge of the counter acting as if he works there, but I know he is pretending.

'But he is a paedophile,' I hiss.

'No, Jen, he isn't. Time to go.' The Norwegian starts to lead me away across the road and back down Woods Parade.

'Jen. It's OK. Don't worry. Nothing bad is going to happen.'

We are half way down the road when I stop and turn to go back.

'I have to do something!'

The Norwegian puts a strong arm around my shoulders turning me back around.

'He is evil, I know it.'

'No, Jen, he isn't.' The Norwegian pulls me into a tight hug. 'Trust me.'

Then a taxi drives past.

'Look a police car!' I say.

'No, Jen, that is a taxi.'

I give him a disbelieving look and start waving at the taxi.

'Jen! It is a taxi.'

Then I remember the security staff from my old school friend's company who are watching over us. *They will catch him. They will know what to do with him.* His company are pulling out all the stops to make sure I'm safe. Barack Obama and me. We are going to use Facebook to get all paedophiles. I am brimming over with joy. I see a huge safety net spanning the world with paedophiles all caught in it and all the children of the world safe. I might even get a knighthood. I know that isn't the point of it, but I think my parents will be so proud of me.

'S'okay,' I say to The Norwegian. 'They will take care of it.'

He smiles me a crooked smile but has stopped asking me what I mean. I let him lead me, and the buggy, back home.

Later that day we sit in the living room: me and The Norwegian, Peter, Clare/Lindsay Lohan and their son Hugo. The Boy is napping in his bassinet. I look at Peter. He is a millionaire, and we didn't even know it. He's kept it hidden so well. He looks relaxed and happy as we sit and chat idly. Something amazing is about to happen. I can tell from the way Peter and Clare/Lindsay seem full to bursting with some exciting news but they aren't ready to tell us yet. If The Norwegian would only shut up and give them the space they need to tell us whatever it is.

I get a flash of inspiration and I know what it is. Peter is going to give my charity, Cerebral Palsy Alliance, one million dollars. He has been so impressed with what I've told him about how the charity is run, and what excellent work we do, he has decided to make his first major gift to our charity. This is amazing. I imagine, after they've told us, ringing my boss, Mike, and putting him on speakerphone so that he can hear for himself. Between us—me, Peter, and the researchers I work with—we really might find a cure for cerebral palsy. We really might. I give Peter a huge smile.

'So, how've you been?' asks Clare/Lindsay.

'It has been very weird and I've had all these strange thoughts. I thought

I was Cameron Diaz earlier this week.'

We all laugh.

'And I thought you were Lindsay Lohan,' I say to Clare/Lindsay. *Still do,* I think.

She almost jumps out of her seat.

'No really!'

'I think I might be part of a group of people who find a cure for cerebral palsy,' I say to Peter. He is leaning back with his hands behind his head. His eyes are brimming with tears. No wonder, giving that much money away to a charity is very emotional.

'And I thought that I was going to be able to use Facebook to catch all,' I pause and my voice catches, '... all paedophiles.'

The Norwegian looks at me sharply. I decide not to say anything about Obama as I don't want to spoil their surprise. My chin sinks to my chest. There is silence until we hear the waking squeaks of The Boy. I get up and go into his room to pick him up.

I'm changing his nappy as I think about Peter the secret millionaire. He must have met Lindsay Lohan in London and fallen in love. Together they relocated to Sydney to get away from the paparazzi. This thought echoes through my consciousness trying to find a place to rest. Peter who always thought people would see the money first and the man second and Clare/Lindsay who had been so traumatised by her child-stardom and crackers parents.

I bring The Boy back into the room as The Norwegian suggests we go for a walk. He keeps talking and won't give Peter the chance he needs to raise the subject. *Come on, be quiet.*

So off we set. The Norwegian and Peter walk ahead and I walk with Clare/Lindsay. I think she'll open up if I let her know that I know about Renée Zellweger being in the building.

'And she's staying with her mum in the ground floor flat of our building.'

'You must write this stuff down,' she says.

'Oh, I will. I'm going to write a book about it.'

As we walk up the path where it joins with Lauderdale Avenue Clare/Lindsay quickly pulls her sunglasses down and sweeps her hair around to cover her face. Poor thing, I think. She's so used to hiding she does it automatically.

As we return from our walk we pass our neighbour's flat.

'This one,' I whisper to Clare/Lindsay. She smiles awkwardly and whisks Peter and Hugo away. No matter, I think, maybe it's best they announce it tomorrow.

And this was one of the better days. On the bad days The Norwegian and I would just argue and argue. One day it was because I thought that he had a photographic memory. The arguments would go on and on, wearing both of us down to exhaustion.

Chapter Fifteen

The Boy is fast asleep and I'm pacing back and forth.

'Something is wrong I just know it.'

'It's OK, Jen. Time for us to go to sleep.'

'One in four children is abused. Did you know that?'

'Yes, you told me.'

I'd been horrified to learn of this statistic at work training. As people with disability are at a higher risk of abuse, everyone who works at the Cerebral Palsy Alliance takes part in training around preventing and responding to abuse.

'One in four,' I say again. As I pace, I go through a list of everyone I know stopping at each fourth person.

'It's so awful. I can hardly stand it.' Tears are streaming down my face. All these friends were abused. How could something so terrible happen?

But then I have a sudden thought that twists my stomach.

'I think I was abused,' I say to The Norwegian.

'I think I may have suppressed the memory.'

'Jen, I don't think so. You are just having lots of strange thoughts at the minute.'

The Norwegian eventually goes to bed and I sit up playing on Facebook.

I wonder if I'll be able to sleep knowing that I'm going to meet Obama tomorrow. For me, the meeting is always tomorrow.

The next day is Sydney special: clear blue sky, the odd puff of cloud and warm balmy temperatures.

The conviction I am going to meet Obama fades. I think back to knowing Peter was going to give us one million dollars and it all seems so unlikely. How can Clare be Lindsay Lohan when she is Clare? The madness and delusions temporarily rinse away leaving me cold and rational.

The day passes with bottles, feeds, nappies and calmness. The Norwegian and I don't argue and everything seems to be returning to normal.

At three o'clock Lautaro comes around and we head out to the North Harbour Reserve to meet some of our friends and their daughter. We kick a football back and forth between us, chat and watch their daughter play on the seesaw.

I spot a dog in the distance and stop speaking mid sentence. The dog is running towards us in great bounds. I frown staring at the dog. I manage to pull myself back from the brink. I can't control dogs with my mind, I think.

'Do you want to sit down?' asks Lautaro. And so we sit on the grass a little away from the others and I carry on telling him about what has been happening.

Sunday turns to Monday and then to Tuesday and despite the upturn on Sunday I get worse and worse with more delusions. One night I think I may have killed a man at university who tried to rape me—another suppressed memory. I spend hours watching De La Soul videos on YouTube.

I write pages and pages of equations and scribbles.

Watch Bridget Jones Diary + Anne of Green Gables + Goodnight Mr Tom + Mr Men + Cranford + Jane Austin + Muppets + Jim Henderson + Eric Carle + Guy Date Chain (choker) + Guy on Table + Boxer + Joe is Christopher Robin = Peter Pan. Sainsbury's = Ginger Guy. May FDP + Olly = Grandpa Jim. Toy Snail + Friends = Magic Roundabout. Being Weird + McDonald's = Dad = Lucky Jim.

$Jim = j + I = m$

$I + j = m$

$m + Castro = I$

Diary of a Wimpy Kid

Sarah + Michael = He is my brother

He ain't heavy

$H + e = I$

Bill is me + William = Bunce

Bill + am = teacher

Jo is my sister

Teffa = Judy 1

Tuffa + Judy 2 = Kath

Kath Kelly + Fred = ?

Our Willy = Oor Wullie

The Browns = Kill

$K + I = Kill\ I\ am$

K Dora = Scrabble

Monopoly + bull bars = Dead kid.

One day I have a mini shopping spree at our local mall in Balgowlah. In a clothes shop I'm convinced that the items for sale are based on treasures rescued from the Titanic. What they don't realise is they have included the original relics by mistake. I am so excited, but don't want to give the game away, riffling through the racks to find the 'original' items, and buying bags and necklaces like they are going out of fashion. It's the same story in the shop next door. I buy some white enamel doorknobs with IN and OUT on them, convinced they are the very door knobs from the kitchens on the Titanic.

That night The Norwegian and I have a marathon argument and I start to experience a feeling like I am not in control of my body. I am terrified about holding The Boy fearing I may drop him if my arms aren't under my control.

Eventually we both lie in bed exhausted. Then The Norwegian starts to cry. My body calms and I kneel next to The Norwegian on the bed holding him tight as he cries and cries.

'I'm so sorry. So sorry,' I say.

He cries on.

'I can't stand the arguing any more,' he says.

'I know. I'm sorry.'

The Norwegian slowly calms down and stops crying. He lies there making small movements. I don't know what he is doing.

'What's happening? Are you OK.'

'I'm just doing that relaxation technique, you know the one, when I tense a part of my body and then relax it.'

'I think you are having a panic attack.'

'No, Jen, I'm doing this on purpose.'

'That's what you think.'

'Please, Jen. Please no more.'

He stops and I lie down next to him holding him tight.

'Have you ever had a panic attack before?'

He is silent and we both eventually drop off into fitful sleep.

The Norwegian has to take another week off work. The Extended Hours Team start talking about options.

'Hospital,' they say, and my heart clamps shut for a second, freezing my blood and closing my chest.

'No, no. I can't go to hospital.'

'It's just an option.'

'I'm going mad,' I sob my hands covering my face. The tears run down my palms.

'No Jen, you've got something caused by pregnancy and the birth. You haven't got schizophrenia. You will get 100% better, this much we know.'

'Really? Really?'

'Yes, without doubt. But you need some help right now.'

'It would be more for me than you, really, Jen. I don't know how much longer I can carry on,' says The Norwegian.

As well as looking after me in my confused, hallucinating, deluded and highly irritable state, The Norwegian had taken most responsibility for looking after The Boy. Trying to keep up with me, and keep on top of things in the house, was taking its toll. We'd had takeaway every night in the last week. I was in such a state I didn't realise how much work The Norwegian was doing just to keep our heads above water.

'We've got you an appointment on Monday with The Doctor. You met him earlier this week. He will assess whether you need to go into hospital or not.'

'Will I get sectioned?' The word echoes around the room. Sectioned. Sectioned. Sectioned.

'Jen, no—you would be a voluntary patient.'

After they leave I start crying again. My eyes are squeezed shut and the tears are building up under my eyelids. I open my eyes and a flood of tears washes my face.

'I can't go to hospital; what am I going to do?'

The Norwegian hugs me close and we get ready for settling The Boy for the night.

Chapter Sixteen

The next day we are sitting in the reception of the adult mental health unit waiting for our appointment with The Doctor. I am clutching a photograph of my sister and me. I know I need it today but I don't know why. The woman behind reception smiles at The Norwegian as he takes The Boy out of his buggy and joggles him on his knee.

A young man of 18 or 19 comes and sits in the reception area. He is looking over at The Boy. I smile at him. He is wearing a grey t-shirt and grey jogging bottoms with flip-flops. He has pink flesh-coloured plasters wrapped around each toe contrasting against his brown skin. He has some tobacco, papers, a lighter and loose change in a clear zip-lock plastic bag. His eyes are wide and he nervously looks away.

'Hello,' I say and his smile flicks on for a moment and then is gone. He reminds me so much of my sister, not in looks, but the way he holds his body slow and still as if waiting for a punch, and the confused, frightened blinking of his eyes.

'I love kids,' he says slowly fumbling the bag. I feel a great surge of protectiveness towards him.

I tell him The Boy's name. The Norwegian smiles over and then goes back to playing with The Boy.

'That's a good name,' the young man says extracting the tobacco and papers. He starts to roll a cigarette. He has schizophrenia. I know it. His hands tremble slightly as he puts the rollie between his lips.

'Nice name,' he says as he stands and starts to walk out the door.

'Hey,' I say, and I hold up the picture of my sister and me. 'You will get better you know.'

He stops and turns back, a big smile transforming his frozen face.

'I just know it,' I say holding the photograph forward so he can see.

'Thanks,' he says pushing the door open and stepping outside. 'Thanks.'

I sit and look at the photograph. Maybe that is why this is happening to me. I'm going to cure schizophrenia. Maybe that's why I'm meeting this senior doctor. With my insight and personal experience, and his knowledge and connections, between us we are going to cure schizophrenia. A bolt of pure happiness passes through me. My sister—I am going to cure her. She can come and live with us in Australia. She is going to get better.

In the picture my arm is around her shoulder. My eyes fill with tears of happiness. I can cure someone by just telling a person they are going to be OK. It is all so clear now. They believe me because I'm right and the placebo effect does the rest. All I need to do is fly back to England and tell my sister she is going to get better and she will.

'It's all going to be OK,' I say to The Norwegian.

He looks up, smiling. 'It's good you feel like that,' he says.

Then one of the workers I had met when I was first referred to the Extended Hours Team, comes to collect us and we enter The Doctor's office.

He is sitting at his desk and turns around to greet us. We file into the room and sit down. The Norwegian manoeuvres the buggy into a corner.

The Doctor gets up to shake our hands. He is a tall man with a close-cropped beard. He is wearing a shirt with thin purple stripes and gold sun cufflinks. He sits back down, looking at me.

'How are you, Jen?' he asks.

'I've been better, to be honest.' I hold out the photograph. 'I know I've got to show you this, but I don't know why? It's my sister.'

'Can you tell me what's been happening,' he asks. And I explain about the man the day before, and the fact that I think I'm going to cure cerebral palsy *and* schizophrenia. I tell him about Cameron Diaz, Lindsay Lohan, the repressed memories of abuse and attempted rape. I also tell them about what I thought was The Norwegian's panic attack, but they don't seem to worry about it.

As I talk The Doctor slumps further and further down in his seat, his hands steepled as he listens with a serious face. He is so low now he is practically lying down in the chair with his legs splayed open. His bottom lip curls over and droops down his chin, the skin under his eyes melts until I can almost see the bone of his cheeks. It looks so funny that I start to laugh.

The Norwegian has been talking and now looks over at me.

'He looks so funny,' I say looking back at The Doctor who is now sitting upright in his chair. Everyone is staring at me, and I feel my eyes starting to shut.

'I'm so tired,' I giggle, looking again at The Doctor. His face must be made of rubber, I think, stifling another giggle. I can feel myself sliding sideways out of the chair. I'm so tired that I drop into sleep. I'm going to fall off, and a great bubble of laughter swells in my chest. Then I remember the young man outside. I open my eyes and sit up on the chair.

'I met a man in the reception and I know he has schizophrenia. How could I know that?'

'Well, this is a mental health unit. It is a good bet that he has schizophrenia or a related illness.'

'He had plasters around his toes.'

They both smile in recognition and I think: *I'm right.*

'I told him he was going to get better.'

'Why?'

'Because he'll believe me and that will make all the difference.'

'But back to you, Jen,' and the questions continue.

By the end of the meeting it is agreed that I will be going to a perinatal mental health unit. This is a special unit specifically for new mums who are having serious mental health problems. We can stay with The Boy, unlike in more traditional units where the mother and baby would be separated. Even The Norwegian can stay with us in the hospital. We are due to be admitted the following day. Hospital. I am going to Hospital. But they very much make it feel like it is our decision, The Norwegian's and mine.

The Hospital

'The Moon is Important.'

My Diary Entry

93

Chapter Seventeen

'I'm going to throw up. Throw up!'

I'm crouched by the side of the bed. We are in the Perinatal Mental Health Unit.

'Here take this,' says one of the nurses. She hands me a sick bag.

'Too small, I need to get to the bathroom.'

'Probably best if you stay here,' she says.

'Help me,' I say to The Norwegian. He grabs my hand and ignoring The Nurse helps me to the en suite bathroom.

Just in time, I kneel by the toilet, heaving and gasping. It feels like the entire contents of my stomach evacuate in a stream of vomit as wide as my open mouth. My stomach heaves three more times before the nausea passes, and I lean back on my heels gulping. I lean forward again with my arm draped around the seat. The Norwegian and The Nurse are standing in the door of the bathroom looking down on me.

We'd arrived earlier in the day, Friday, with bags packed for a week's stay.

It's a long weekend and everyone we pass on the way to the hospital seems to be bustling along, packing their cars with beach chairs and Frisbees in preparation. We have no such frisson of future pleasure expected.

In the car on the way over The Norwegian is quiet.

'You OK?' I ask.

'I was just about to ask you the same thing. You're very quiet.'

'I'm shitting myself. This is my biggest fear writ large.'

'You are strong, I am strong and you are not going mad.'

'Thank you.' There is a pause. 'God, I made you say that so many times.'

'I know. But it's true. That's why I kept saying it.'

I sit in the car and think about how scared I am about being in a mental hospital. I imagine padded cells and straightjackets.

We arrive at a long, low building and are shown to our room. It is just outside the staff room so, if it is anything like the hospital where The Boy was born, we are going to have disturbed nights. Or, even more disturbed nights than you get with an eight-week old baby.

The Norwegian unpacks while I sit on the bed playing with The Boy. The room is clean and sparsely furnished; a double bed, wardrobe, rocking chair and change table, all plain and sturdy. The little en suite has a walk-in shower, basin and toilet. There are thin but clean white towels folded over a towel rail.

It is twelve o'clock so we decide to head upstairs to the dining room for lunch. My unit is one of many at the hospital and the dining room is starting to fill up with other patients. I scan the room and wonder about the stories of all these people. I see a young girl, painfully thin, with her mother and sister. I see an older man with a wide face and big square glasses sitting on his own. There are two other mothers in the room with their buggies drawn up next to their tables. They must be from my ward.

We fill up on soup, a selection of salads and a roll. The salads are 'serve yourself' from a metal unit on wheels, the compartments of salads lit by an overhead lamp. One of the salads has a funny taste so, after eating a few mouthfuls, I push it to the side.

I think back to that salad while I'm hanging off the toilet seat.

'Food poisoning,' I say unable to manage the demands of proper sentence structure.

'Most likely this is linked to your psychosis,' says The Nurse.

'Really?' says The Norwegian. They both stand there looking at me.

'I think the worst of it is out,' I say.

'Come on, Jen.' The Norwegian holds out his hand, helps me to my feet, then guides me back to bed.

As I lie on the bed my arms and legs start to spasm.

'I'm not in control of my body,' I whisper through clenched teeth. The Norwegian crouches down by the side of the bed holding my hands.

'It is going to be OK,' he says.

The room is contracting and releasing.

'I'm going,' I say.

'You are safe here. I'm here. Everything is going to be OK,' says The Norwegian. But as the room contracts and releases then fades to nothing, the double bed disappears and I realise I am kneeling next to a hard thin mattress on a canvas cot. My hands are clasped together. I am praying. Tears are streaming down my face.

'Please forgive me Lord,' I say. I am looking up at a crucifix through a blur of tears. I feel soiled and dirty. I get to my feet and lift the heavy material of my cassock above my head. I am standing naked by the washstand.

Back in the room, The Nurse and The Norwegian watch my arms and legs jerking and twitching.

I sluice my face with water, then wash under my arms and between my legs. I feel a penis limp and rubbery between my hands.

Why would God test me like this? Why would he put so much temptation in my path? I try to block the images of kissing him, his stubble rough on my lips, his tongue, his hands on my hips pulling me close. How can something so full of the worst sin feel so full of beauty? I thought my love for him was the love of a fellow brother monk, until this morning when a few minutes of weakness had lead me to commit one of the worst sins imaginable. How can I go on here at the monastery?

I roughly dry myself and pull my cassock back over my head. I return to my spot on the floor by the cot and start to pray again. It must all be part of God's plan for me. He is testing my faith, knowing I will fail, to teach me humility. God is good, he loves me but hates my sin. I lean forward with my head resting on my clasped hands. I continue to pray and I can feel the cold floor chilling my knees and shins through my cassock.

The room shimmers and warps again and I realise I can see The Norwegian kneeling close to me.

'I'm OK,' I say.

'Where did you go?'

I point up at the corner of the ceiling.

'There, I went there.'

Chapter Eighteen

The next morning, on Saturday, I have an appointment with one of the GPs attached to the unit. They are worried about my involuntary movements and want me to get a physical health check. We file into the room and put The Boy in his buggy next to the seats. A middle-aged round man with round glasses and a round stomach is sitting at the desk. There is a young Asian man sitting beside him. We take up the other two seats in the room. There is an examining couch in the corner.

'Hello. I understand you've been having some difficulties?'

'Yes,' I smile at him then look pointedly at the young man.

'This is a student who will be observing. You are OK with that?'

'No problem.'

There is a pause.

'So tell me what has been going on with you physically? I've read your notes so you don't need to worry about filling me in on your mental health. I'm here to help with what is going on physically.'

'I've been having some involuntary body movements. There are times when I don't feel in control of my body, which is scary enough, but it makes me very apprehensive about holding our son. I don't want to drop him.'

'Indeed.' He takes my hand and leans forward holding up an instrument.

'I'm just going to check your eyes,' he says shining a small light into my left eye. He flicks the light from one eye to the other while firing questions at me. I try and fire back the answers, keeping up with him.

'How old are you?'

'36.'

'What is your son's birthday?''

'28th January, 2012'

'Who is the Prime Minister?'

'Julia Gillard.'

'Where do you live?'

'Sydney.'

'Where are you now?'

'Perinatal mental health unit,' I say, then 'Oh, shit,' I say as my right arm spasms. He stops smiling and looks down at my arm. Then my left arm spasms, more violently, jerking my hand almost up to shoulder height. It is like I am a puppet, arms yanked by invisible string.

'Oh, God,' I moan. 'What's happening to me?'

'Let's get you lying down.' He takes my arm in a firm grip and leads me to the examining couch. A huge spasm ripples through my whole body and my knees give way. The doctor catches me and The Norwegian jumps up from his seat to take my other hand. They both lie me down on the examining couch.

'So frightened,' I whisper. I have my eyes closed as one last spasm rips through me and then it is over. I lie on my back staring up at the ceiling waiting for my heart to slow, my breathing to regulate.

'What do you know about Tourettes?'

'Tourettes?'

'Yes.'

'Swearing, I guess.'

'Anything else?'

'Do you think I have Tourettes?' I ask incredulously.

'No, I'm just trying to rule out certain conditions. I don't think you have Tourettes, or epilepsy. You remained conscious while you were having the involuntary movements. If you had epilepsy you wouldn't do that.'

'Good news, I suppose.' I go to sit up.

'Whoa there, Jennifer, just relax on your back for a minute.'

'Jen, call me Jen. So what do you think it is, then?'

'Most likely it is part of your mixed episode, part of your psychosis.'

'Weird.' I say.

'Weird?'

'Well I was thinking about the mood stabilisers. It is a bit strange that I start taking an epilepsy drug and then start having fits.'

'Well, no, not fits. As I said you'd need to be unconscious for us to consider epilepsy. I can reassure you that you don't have epilepsy.'

I smile with relief, but the doubt remains. It just seems like too much of a coincidence. I wonder what they are trying to hide from me. Why would they lie?

'Sodium valproate is a very effective mood stabiliser. That is why you are taking it.'

I turn to smile at The Norwegian. In the fluoro light of the small room he looks pale and drawn with dark smudges under his eyes. But he smiles back at me.

'I feel a bit better now. I think I can get up.'

* * *

Those turn out to be the last of the involuntary body movements. I never find out why they happened or why they stopped. We also find out that some of the other patients and staff had vomiting, so it is extremely unlikely that my vomiting was part of my psychosis, though none of the staff acknowledge this.

* * *

One of the hard things about mental health problems is they tend to overshadow physical problems. If you think you are Cameron Diaz it is easy for other people to dismiss the things you are saying, for example, that you have a terrible headache or backache. This phenomenon is known as 'diagnostic overshadowing', where the fact a person has a mental health diagnosis can cause GPs and other health professionals to focus less on the person's physical health.

My sister has struggled in the past to get some of her team of supporters to recognise her physical difficulties. Her last two relapses have been triggered by physical problems: a really bad toothache caused by years of neglect, and back pain caused by over-vigorous digging in her allotment. Both times, being in pain and needing someone around to help her, brought home how alone she is, leading to feelings of sadness, and then to not taking her meds. Luckily, the current team looking after Jo, really understand her and caught the bad-back relapse early. This meant she could go into a halfway house for intensive support rather than back to the psychiatric unit of the local hospital. She is in the halfway house now, slowly building up her confidence to live independently again.

* * *

After the doctors, I have a rest in our room while The Norwegian mixes a bottle and feeds The Boy. They are sitting on the wooden rocking chair rocking backwards and forwards. The Norwegian smiles down at The Boy. We have a canteen lunch of beer-battered fish and chips, skipping the salad this time, then we decide to go for an explore of the local area.

We discover the local park a few minutes stroll away from the hospital. This beautiful green space is modelled on the Union Jack. The whole park is a rectangle with paths representing both the upright cross and the diagonal cross. In the centre of the two crosses, in the middle of the park, is a large bandstand occupied by a trio of legging-clad women doing shoulder stands on their yoga mats. As we stroll through in the afternoon sunshine we watch an elegant pair of Chinese women doing the slow and controlled movement of Tai Chi. Footballs and Frisbees are being kicked and thrown, and a group of Chinese or Korean men play a game like volleyball but with a small wicker ball. I think it is the most beautiful park I've ever seen.

We are seated on one of the benches overlooking the playing field.

'I've had two amazing ideas,' I say.

'Yeah?'

'I'm going to set up a Local Park Appreciation Society.'

'Sounds good,' The Norwegian smiles at me.

'Also, I think the moon's gravitational pull affects our brains very slightly. I think this will be the key factor in finding a cure for schizophrenia—they always knew there was a link between the moon and madness, hence the word lunatic, luna meaning moon.'

There is a pause, then he says, 'Interesting.'

'God, you are so sarcastic. You could just try to believe me.'

He bends his head forward and slowly rubs his face with his hands.

'I need a time out,' I snap. 'I'll take The Boy back to the hospital and you can stay here.'

'OK.' His voice is flat and he won't meet my eyes.

'I'm the one that's ill you know; you could try and be more considerate.'

* * *

One of the toughest things to come to terms with throughout this period is how hard things were for The Norwegian. Being so wrapped up in layers of mania and madness I just didn't see how much he was struggling and how selfish I was being. Unbeknown to me, The Norwegian was starting to crack under the strain of seeing the one he loved so changed. Over the next few days he would walk to the park on his own and sit on a bench and just cry. His hope that a stay at the hospital would make things better was wearing thin—I was still argumentative and highly irritable. The arguments were very repetitive where I would get angry if he didn't go along with my delusions. The worst was when he felt I was attacking his personality, saying he was weak and not able to support me properly.

* * *

I storm back, pushing the buggy fast through the residential streets surrounding the hospital. When I get back, one of the nurses sees me as I push open the door to our room. She has large, doleful eyes, a puffed-up squashy face and short brown hair.

'Where have you been?'

'For a walk.'

'On your own?'

'Yes, for some of it.'

'You are not allowed out unescorted.'

'What! No one told me. Why?'

'You are coming out of psychosis.'

'But I'm a voluntary patient so how can I not be allowed out?'

'You can if you're escorted. It is just to be safe.'

* * *

My sister has spent years of her life in locked wards where she wasn't allowed out unescorted. She has been effectively locked up for years, in what is as close to prison as you can get, without committing any crime, against her will and with no idea how long her 'sentence' is. When she is very ill this is the best place, as well as the worst place, for her. If you are paranoid and delusional it is very hard to take, being watched all the time. And it doesn't help if your fellow inmates are just as unhinged (if not more so) than you.

A sane person locked up in a psych ward, would shout and scream to be let out. All through her worst periods, Jo would think she was fine and beg and plead to be let out. The security is tight on locked wards. They often have an 'airlock' system to get in and out, with two sets of doors. Before entering, you are given a locker to store forbidden items like matches or lighters. They open one door and you enter the airlock, the first door is locked behind you before the second door opens.

Once she starts getting better, in any of the wards she's been on, she is given more and more freedom; going out escorted with two members of staff at first, then just one, then with family and, finally, on her own.

The first time she was in hospital for 18 months, but after the first three months, she was trusted and given some more freedom. I was walking home from school after my GCSE maths exam and, for once, not thinking about my sister. I was planning the revision I would do that afternoon and thinking about my technology exam in two day's time.

When I got home and opened the gate, I saw my sister waiting on the front doorstep of our home, 106 Osbaldeston Road. I stopped, standing motionless and stared up at her.

'I've come home,' she said. 'I don't want to be in hospital any more.'

She sat leaning against the black-painted door, the brass knocker and figures one, zero and six above her head.

'Are you OK?' I asked.

'Hungry.'

I fished my keys out of the side pocket of my school bag and opened the door.

'Hello, there!' called Helen, our cleaner. Helen came to the house every day to polish, iron, vacuum and dust. She was also there so I had someone to come home to before Mum and Dad returned from work.

'Hi Helen, Jo's here,' I called up the stairs. There was a sudden silence as the vacuum cleaner was switched off. Then Helen came down the stairs. Jo walked past me and down into the kitchen. I stood in the hall clutching my school bag. Helen walked towards me.

'You OK?' she asked.

'I'll try and get hold of Mum,' I whispered. She nodded and went into the kitchen. I heard her cheery voice while she chatted to Jo. I raced up the stairs to the study and pulled the address book out of the shelf by the phone. I dialled Mum's direct line at Hackney College. It rang through to the voicemail.

'Mum, it's Jen, Jo's here. Can you come home?'

I put down the phone and sat waiting for a second, willing it to ring back and be Mum saying she would take care of everything. I searched through the address book to see if the main switchboard number was there. Remember this was before mobiles and Google. I tried again and it went through to voicemail again. A big sob gulped up from my stomach.

'Any luck?' said Helen, standing in the study doorway.

'No. Voicemail.'

'Don't worry Jen, it'll be all right.' She came in and put her hand on my shoulder.

'She attacked Mum last week.'

'Did she? I'm so sorry.'

'Grabbed her hair and dragged her to the ground.'

I tried the number again and this time Mum picked up.

'She's here. Jo's here.'

'Don't worry, I'll be straight home.'

'But what if she attacks you again.'

There was silence.

'It'll be OK, don't worry,' she said eventually. 'You sit tight, I'll be back in 20 minutes.'

I hung up and slowly made my way down the stairs into the kitchen.

Jo had her back to me and turned as she heard me enter the room. In her right hand she was holding a large knife. Her face was blank. I stood still looking at her, holding my breath. The late afternoon light glinted on the blade. A hot flash of fear shot through me. *Is she going to stab me?* I tried a smile. It was a pathetic attempt, too wide, too bright with teeth showing.

A slow smile crept onto her face.

'Sandwich?' she asked going back to the loaf on the kitchen counter in front of her. She sawed back and forth through the crust and the soft middle of the bread.

That moment right there, right there when I thought she might stab me, was one of the worst of my life. She didn't want to stab me, she was just making a sandwich. I felt the guilt soak through me. She had never, and has never threatened me or shouted at me, not like she does sometimes with

Mum and Dad. She always treated me well, even when she was really unwell.

'Jo, what are you doing here?'

She turned back to me, the bread forgotten for the moment.

'I want to come home. It's horrible in the hospital. I don't feel safe there. I'm not ill any more. I'm better. I don't hear voices.'

'Hospital is the best place for you now.'

'That's just Mum talking. I know that. I know Mum doesn't want me back. That's because she is a vampire. That's why me and you are baby vampires.'

'Mum's not a vampire, Jo.'

She rolled her eyes and turned to the fridge. She took out butter, cheese and ham, and placed them next to the sliced bread.

'Dad's a saint. You know that right? He breathes for me.'

'When you say things like that you don't sound better.'

She layered the cheese and ham onto the bread and flipped the second slice on top.

'I can't stay in hospital. It's so bad.'

'I know it is tough but you are ill.'

'If I'm ill then I should be with my family.'

I gave up and went to get a glass from the cupboard. A key scrabbled in the lock of the front door.

'I'm home,' said Mum.

Jo looks towards the front door, her face contorted with hatred.

'Vampire,' she whispers.

'I'll just clear up, shall I?' I said stepping forward. I scooped up the knife and breadboard and put them in the sink out of reach.

'I'm going to my room,' said Jo, as Mum entered the kitchen.

'Jo, I have to take you back.'

'I'm not going.'

'It is for the best.'

'What do you know?' She stomped downstairs to her room in the basement. Her sandwich lay forgotten on the counter top. Mum came over to me and held my hand.

'Are you OK?'

'Yeah, I'm fine. I was a bit—' I started crying.

'I thought she was going to stab me.'

Mum held me tight until my sobs lessened.

'Oh, Jen.' she said.

* * *

Now I am a mother I know all she wanted to do was make things OK for me and for my sister, but in the face of the devastation of schizophrenia there was almost nothing she could do. It is a tough lesson to learn at 15, that things can go so wrong and stay wrong. *It'll all be OK*, the comforting words of a mother to a child, would have been a lie and had no place with us on that day.

* * *

Mum, the brave woman that she is, managed to get Jo in the car and back safely to the ward. After they left I went up to my room and looked at my technology folder. I sat at the desk reading through my notes failing in my efforts to memorise the definition of a nanofarad. The words on the paper were jumbled, jumping over each other. I leant forward and rested my forehead on the cool pages. But I sat up before the tears had a chance to drip onto the paper and smudge the words. I needed to be able to read them if I was going to get any revision done.

* * *

Back in my own room I am starting to get a taste of what it must have been like for my sister over the years, just a taste, as here I have much more freedom than she had, but still the restrictions chafe.

We find out later that starting our stay at the beginning of a long weekend is less than ideal as they have a skeleton staff and most of the senior people are away. This explains the curious lack of attention even though I am being watched. No one comes to tell me what is going to happen, how things work and what is expected of me. They have a watch and wait brief with me.

I stomp upstairs to get lunch and place The Boy in his pushchair next to me. I am ravenous and polish off a huge plate of chicken curry, rice and poppadoms. At this stage, along with all the other things they hadn't told us, they also hadn't discussed the side effects of the medication I was taking. I now know that olanzapine is well known for sedation and weight gain; it makes you very hungry. It may not be so serious, but weight gain can impact hugely on anyone's self-confidence, especially if you are already depressed and anxious.

But, as I didn't know this, I was eating for England ... I've always been able to eat whatever I want and not really put on weight, as long as I do exercise, but the olanzapine dramatically alters my metabolism as well as making me starving hungry. I put on five kilos in two weeks, adding to the extra five kilos I put on while I was pregnant. At first I think my clothes have shrunk, I really do. As soon as they tell me about the side effect I'm able to stop eating so much and my weight levels out at 75 kg, 10 kg heavier than my pre-pregnant self.

After lunch I find The Norwegian lying on the bed with his eyes closed. I shut the door behind me.

'Now they are telling me I'm not allowed to go out on my own.'

'Really?'

'What are they going to do about it if I do? They can't fucking-well watch me every moment. They won't even know I'm gone.'

He lets out a huge sigh.

'Sorry about earlier,' I say.

'S'okay. I'm just so tired.'

I sit next to him on the bed and stroke his arm.

'I just need you to believe me more.'

'But Jen, some of the stuff you are saying is so out there. It is like when you thought that man was a paedophile; you knew it wasn't right the next day. I can't agree with stuff I know is wrong, can I? But you get so mad at me.'

We sit in silence.

'But what if I'm right and the moon—'

'No, Jen, no more.'

Later that afternoon I go into the patients' kitchen to sterilise The Boy's bottles. As I slosh water around in the bottles, thoughts about breastfeeding swirl around my head. I am still desperate to breastfeed. No one understands how much it matters to me. The staff just blithely assumed I would stop with no thought to the emotional repercussions. *Surely I'll not be on the medication for long. As long as I continue to stimulate my breasts I can go back to breastfeeding.*

* * *

No one explains that I'll need to keep taking the medication for months, if not years. I suppose knowing that could have made me more upset, and that's why they didn't tell me. Maybe, as they knew I'd be on medication long-term, they just assumed I would somehow know this too. Or they all assumed someone else, someone more up to speed with my situation, would have explained it to me. Or, perhaps they didn't put that much thought into it—it seeming so obvious to an outsider that halting breastfeeding was the only sensible option.

* * *

The Norwegian and I argue fiercely over breastfeeding. He tries to convince me that it is OK to stop and I accuse him of not understanding how much it means to me. He finds out that, according to the Australian Breastfeeding Association, 92% of children are breastfed at birth, falling to 56% at three months, and only 14% at six months.

Looking back, I still don't understand why this was such a big deal for me as I genuinely believe that bottle-feeding is no problem, as some women, for many different reasons, just can't breastfeed.

I think it had something to do with control. Being a new mum and learning to care for a baby is a lesson in learning to live with chaos. There was so much in my life that was out of my control, especially being ill, I probably just wanted something to work the way 'it was supposed to.'

* * *

The kitchen is small and neat with rows of cabinets and a double sink along one wall, and a fridge and shelf with a row of sterilisers on the other. One of the other patients is feeding her daughter purée. She turns to me and says hello. She has short fair hair standing up in tufts around her head and widely-spaced, blue eyes.

'And how old is this little cutie?' I ask.

'Nine months.'

'Wow, she's a good eater.'

I turn to the sterilisers and open one to put in the bottles. I fill up the little reservoir with water and press the steam button.

'Hi.'

'Nice to meet you.'

'What are you in for?' she asks.

I laugh.

'That makes it sound like prison.'

'But it is like prison here. I call us the inmates rather than patients.'

'I've only just been admitted two days ago.'

'I've been here for weeks; this is my third stay.'

'I'm sorry to hear that.'

'I want to leave but they won't let me.' There is the silence and she turns back to her daughter ladling spoonfuls of thick orange purée from a round Tupperware pot.

'What's that?' she says to her daughter. 'This is yummy, isn't it? I know you like this one. You're such a good girl. Yes you are.'

She wasn't doing anything that a thousand mothers haven't done talking to their babies; holding a one sided conversation. But there was something about the way she held her head to one side, as if really listening, that reminded me of my sister, Jo.

* * *

When Jo was living in a hospital in Aylesbury, I went to visit her one weekend. We were having a café lunch in the market square when a man walked passed with a little puppy on a lead. Jo jumped up, leaving behind her egg and bacon sandwich and mug of tea, and ran over to the dog. Crouching down next to it she said:

'Hello, you little thing. Aren't you cute?'

The owner smiled indulgently.

'Yes you are, yes you are.' She continued patting the little dog on its head.

'You're such a good dog. I know. I know.'

By now the owner was getting a little uncomfortable; Jo hadn't looked up at him or acknowledged him in any way.

* * *

I know that, on some level, Jo really thought the dog was communicating with her. It was not as extreme as hearing a voice, but was some way of 'knowing' what the dog was thinking. As I sensed that then, I'm pretty sure now, that my fellow 'inmate' thinks her baby is really communicating with her.

'I have postpartum psychosis,' I say. 'That's what I'm in for.'

She turns to me.

'Me too.'

We both look at each other in silence. Third visit, I think, and my heart freezes.

The baby starts calling for some more food with a soft burble.

Suddenly, my fellow PPP survivor starts talking in a rapid stream, words tumbling out of her mouth as she tells me what has been happening to her. She is speaking so fast I can hardly keep up. I finish the bottles but don't know how to end the conversation.

'The second time I was admitted she was six-months, and I was in a terrible state. I thought that the government was spying on me. I know that they weren't, but they were, too, at the same time, if that makes sense.'

In a strange way it sort of did.

'Nice to meet you. I've got to ...' I point at the door. She stops talking and wipes her daughter's sticky fingers with the kitchen sponge.

'See you in Group this afternoon?' she says as I leave the kitchen.

As I walk back to our room I see one of the nurses.

'What's Group?' I ask.

'Oh we don't think you are ready for Group yet.'

'But what is it?'

'The patients come together and talk about their experiences with a facilitator. You need to settle in a bit more first.'

'Another thing it would have been nice to know about,' I say.

She looks at me with her lips drawn together.

Chapter Nineteen

The next day, Sunday, The Norwegian is with The Boy in the room and I go for an explore. In the middle of the confusing corridors, hallways and rooms I find a central courtyard. It has two large trees and mature plantings. It lies off a large wooden porch, which houses a small kiosk serving coffee and cakes. It is so peaceful, so calm. It was probably a courtyard when the building was a monastery. I think back to my monk delusions and imagine the monks coming to the courtyard for prayer and quiet meditation. I see ghosts of figures tending to the plants, watering, and sitting on the old benches.

I sit reading my book as the friendly, chirpy young woman behind the counter greets and acknowledges the people who come to see her and fill up on coffee and cakes, tea and biscuits. When the queue dies down she pulls out a chair at the table next to me and sits down for a second.

'What are you reading?' she asks and we chit chat about my book until another person comes to the kiosk for their coffee. She is the first person I've spoken to who treats me just like an ordinary person, not a collection of vexing symptoms. I smile as she bobs her dark head behind the coffee machine.

Suddenly something catches my eye in the tree. I see an amazing bird. I have never seen anything like it before. It looks like half a bird, half a lizard. It has a long fine neck and slim rounded head. Its feathers are short and glisten like scales in the morning sunshine. I watch as it jumps from branch to branch. I finish my tea and go back to the room.

'It's so nice in the courtyard.' I say.

'Yes I went and had a coffee there yesterday when you said you wanted time out,' says The Norwegian.

I can't keep on saying sorry but I do.

'Sorry.'

'Jen, it's OK, but I think it is a good idea for us to have some time apart. I can look after The Boy and you can have a break.'

'When do you get a break?'

He laughs.

'I'm not joking.'

'Jen, I—'
'Why do you always have to have the last word?'
'I don't. It's just—'
'See, you can't just leave it.'
'You asked me a question.'
'I know, and you just had to answer it.'
'What else could I do?'
'You just don't understand.'
'You're right. I really don't.'
'See I told you.'

There is a silence. He is looking at me; grief, annoyance and concern are layered through his face. I know he wants to say something—to have the last word. But then I realise that is the wrong way around. He always makes *me* have the last word.

'I'll be back,' I say. 'They still haven't given me my meds this morning.'

I leave the room and go to the staff room. As usual the door is shut and the sign says 'Handover In Progress.' I look through the glass. It doesn't look like a handover. Two nurses I don't recognise are sitting chatting idly, while a third studies a manila folder of notes. They could even be my notes, for all I know. I wait, hanging around outside trying to catch someone's eye. No luck, and in the end I knock loudly. This place is really starting to get to me. A nurse comes to the door.

'Yes?'
'My meds. I haven't had them yet.'
'Oh, yes, we were just about to come around.'
'I'm pretty sure I shouldn't have to remind you about my meds.' The other two nurses in the room look up at the tone of my voice. One looks briefly at the other. I wonder if I'm starting to get a reputation for being 'difficult'.

'I assume it is a good idea to take them promptly at the same time each day? Or am I wrong.'

'No, you're right, but we were just about to come around.' She is as bad as The Norwegian always having to have the last word.

'Were you doing a handover?' I can't help myself.
'What?'
'It says so on the door.'
She looks at me with a wrinkled brow.

'Let's get your meds then, shall we?' she says with a bright, false smile. She reaches back towards her desk and picks up a bunch of keys. I stand next to her as she opens up the meds trolley. This is a small portable desk-like piece of furniture on wheels. She unlocks the top flap and reveals cubbyholes filled with white boxes with printed labels on them.

She gets out my meds and I take them. Just like that. I wonder what they do with people who are resistant to taking their meds. I walk back to the room. The Norwegian is just settling The Boy for a nap. I sit on the bed.

'This place is starting to get to me.'

He looks at me, trying to assess if he is 'allowed' to reply.

'You and me both.'

When The Boy wakes, The Norwegian and I decide to set off for the local mall. The day before, when we were walking to the park, we noticed a swimming pool attached to the local private school.

'I wonder if I could go swimming there?' I'd said.

'Let's go in and see.'

We wandered in and found out that the pool isn't open to the public, but I could come and have a swimming lesson if I liked.

'But I don't have my cossie here,' I said to The Norwegian.

'We could go to the mall and get you one.'

So now I am guiding the buggy out of our room and past the staff room. I know, now, that I need to tell people if I'm going off site so I knock on the door, despite the 'Handover' sign still being displayed.

'Just off to do a spot of shopping.'

'Are you going to the mall?' asks The Nurse.

'Yes.' I prickle with annoyance. Maybe this is another thing I'm not supposed to do.

'I don't know if that is such a good idea.' I wait. She continues 'I find it's like a long dark tunnel with people coming at you; all streaming out, all looking the same.'

'Oh, well, my husband will be with me so I'm sure it will be OK.'

As we walk through the park to the local mall I tell The Norwegian what The Nurse said.

'Does make you wonder which one of you has mental health problems, if she thinks that,' he says. I grip his hand.

When we get to the mall, it doesn't remotely look like a long tunnel, but it is very busy. Most of the other shoppers are Asian: Chinese, Korean and Taiwanese.

We decide to split up and meet again in two hours at the café in the entrance to the mall. I then go on the biggest spending spree of my life. Normally, I hate shopping: I drag myself around the shops and, even if I really need something, I have great difficulty actually buying it. But today, my normal hesitation disappears and the wonders of the mall open up to me like a jewelled box of treasures.

I spend over $1,000 in one day. At Lorna Jane I buy two yoga pants and a top, a box of socks, headband, two bikinis and one sports bra. I chat to the sales assistant about Lorna Jane the person; she is so inspirational and makes clothes that are exactly what I want. I decide I am going to write a book about her, and her inspirational story.

At David Jones I can barely contain my excitement. I buy two expensive jumpers, a Country Road bag, a Ladybird notebook and pack of rainforest playing cards. At Diva I buy three necklaces, five pairs of earrings, two rings and another headband. In a surf shop I buy a bright blue wristwatch for $10. Bargain. I enjoy the shopping like never before. It seems like a deeply meaningful activity. The things I buy are like missing parts of my soul. I feel with these clothes, bags and jewellery I can make myself whole again.

* * *

Overspending is a classic symptom of mania. People with long-term or reoccurring mania can get themselves into serious debt. My mania was still strong in the first few days, hence all the arguments with The Norwegian.

* * *

I meet The Norwegian at the appointed time laden down with plastic bags full of my treasure.

'I found so many good things, this mall is amazing,' I say as we order, a skim flat white for The Norwegian and an English breakfast tea for me.

The Norwegian looks at my pile of bags and says nothing, tucking the worry away with all the others. Luckily, we had saved up a fair amount to cope with going down to one salary while I was on maternity leave, and the spending doesn't put us into the red.

After my shopping success we head back to the hospital. I had noticed a sign for art therapy earlier so, after a lunch of beef casserole and mash, I leave The Norwegian with The Boy and head for the art therapy room which is through two dark double doors and at the end of a long upwardly slanting corridor.

There are two people waiting to go in. One woman with black straight hair and huge dark eyes, and a large square man with square glasses who I'd seen in the dining room on our first day in hospital.

'Hello,' I say to the woman. 'Is this for art therapy?'

'Yes. Your first time?'

'Yep.'

'Well, you're in for a treat,' she smiles at me.

By the time the two staff members arrive there are 10 or so people waiting, leaning against the wall or sitting on the floor of the corridor outside the room. One of the staff opens the door and we file inside. The room is amazing. It has one wall of storage with drawings and paintings stuck to the doors of the cupboards. The art is a riot of colour and textures. One catches my eye— a picture of a brain with arrows pointing. Words on the page say, 'Art is a way for the brain to heal itself.' I feel all the art materials calling out to me. The room hums with energy and everyone is vibrating too.

The counter, running around two sides of the room, is full of boxes with every type of art material you can imagine. There are palettes and tubes of paint; and boxes and boxes of coloured pencils, charcoal and chalk; and miniature chests of draws filled with beads and jewellery-making materials. We all cluster around a table in the middle of the room. A young woman opposite me gets out a half-finished drawing. It is of a phoenix rising from flames. The flames seem to flicker and dance on the page.

'That's good,' I say to her. She smiles, nods and goes back to drawing the flames in orange pencil.

A clean sheet of paper is calling out particularly strongly so I get up and carefully pick it up and place it on the table in front of my seat. It is so clean, white and unblemished. It seems almost criminal to mark its virginal beauty. My hand hovers over a pencil jar filled with markers, crayons and pencils. They are vibrating at different frequencies. One is still amongst the humming, whirling mass and I carefully slide it out of the jar. It is a blue marker pen with a thick nib.

I start to draw. Sweeps and curls of blue fill the paper in front of me. I pick up a handful of plaster of Paris shells from a container on the counter behind me and hunt down some glue. As I am sticking the shells to the paper I notice the woman with the dark eyes is quietly crying. As I look at her, the room shifts slightly and stops humming. She and the woman next to her are making jewellery. She is holding a thin metal loop and stringing beads onto it as the tears roll down her face.

'I miss them so much,' she says. Her friend is sitting quietly by her side looking at the beads she has collected in front of her. I look about and the two staff members are engrossed with two other patients and their art. I get up and stand next to one of the art therapists. She looks up at me with her eyebrows raised.

'Do you have any tissues?' I whisper, motioning towards the crying woman.

'Yes, of course,' she says handing them to me. To my surprise she doesn't go over to the woman in tears.

I sit back down and hand the tissue box to the woman. Her friend smiles at me.

'Are you OK?' I ask. She smiles through her tears.

'I thought I was going home today. But they tell me I can't.'

'I'm sorry.'

'It's my daughter's birthday tomorrow, and I thought I'd be out of here. I'm making this for her.' She holds up the small bracelet.

'How old?'

'Nine. And my eldest is eleven.'

There is a pause. She looks at my drawing.

'I like that,' she says and she smiles again. I carry on creating swirls and loops and think about my illness and how long it might last. I wonder if I'll still need medication, or hospital, when The Boy is nine. The thought chills me. I look down at my drawing and start to panic. The walls suddenly seem to threaten inwards with their claustrophobic piles of clutter. I start to get to my feet when one of the art therapists sits down next to me.

'I like this,' she says.

'Oh, thanks. They're sort of doodles really.'

'I like your mix of materials: paper, pen and plaster of Paris. Very creative.'

I smile at her and the feeling of panic fades.

The hour draws to a close and we all start packing up our art. Pencils and chalk go back into the cluster of pencil boxes in the middle of the table. The man with square glasses turns the canvas he'd been working on to show one of the staff members. It is an abstract landscape with an orange swirl for a sun and twisted, purple gum trees.

'You've managed to capture the calm before the thunderstorm,' the therapist says to him. He smiles and props the canvas on the counter to dry.

I get up to leave as I've done my packing away.

'I hope you get to leave soon,' I say to the dark-eyed woman as I duck out the door.

* * *

Again, that night, dinnertime passes and they still haven't given me my meds. Last night we'd tried an experiment to see if they would totally forget if we didn't nag them for it. They did eventually come with a handful of tablets, but I'd already fallen asleep and The Norwegian had to wake me up.

I go to the staff room. As usual the door is shut and the 'Handover In Progress' sign is up. This time I don't wait around to see if I can catch someone's eye and just knock straight away. The Nurse comes to the door.

'Meds?'

'Oh, yes, give me a minute.' She grabs her keys from the desk and steps to the medication cabinet in the corridor. She flips open the doors and starts riffling through the boxes of medication.

'Right, so what do we need for you?' she asks.

'Don't you know? It should be on my notes.'

She sighs.

'Yes, it will be in your notes but it's a good idea if you also know what medication you are taking.'

'I have it written down. I don't know it off by heart. I could get my notebook?'

'No, that's fine; I'll just check your notes.' She goes back into the staff room to get my notes and then comes back and picks up three boxes from the cabinet. She pops pills out of blister packs and hands them to me in a small paper cup.

'Why do I have to keep reminding you about my meds?'

The Nurse sighs again.

'It is just, if I wasn't being compliant, I'd be missing my meds, wouldn't I?'
'We shouldn't have to remind you.'
'Well, I feel I shouldn't have to remind you!'

She is being impossible. Always having to have the last word. Just like The Norwegian earlier. Why does everyone want to argue with me?

'There you go,' she says.
'Oh, and by the way, was a handover in progress?'
'What?'
'Well, the sign on the door says 'Handover In Progress', but it is always up.'
'Jen, how are you feeling?'
'I'm fine, really; just getting frustrated with how things are run here.'
'You just need to give it time. Things will come right in a few days when the medication has had a chance to kick in properly.'

She looks at me with concern in her eyes. She can't accept that I might have legitimate reasons to complain. She sees me only as a woman with a mental health problem and not as someone who might have real reasons to be annoyed. I let her have the last word and wonder what observation about my state of mind she might record on my notes. Perhaps, *Jen is highly irritable and resisting taking ownership of her medication.*

* * *

The next morning, Monday, we are walking out of the ward to go to my swimming lesson. I have a bag packed with one of my brand new bikinis, towel and goggles. We walk past The Nurse in the corridor.

'Where are you going?' she asks.
'Swimming,' I say.
'We need you to do a blood test. Can you go later?'
'But I have a swimming lesson booked.'
'A lesson!'

I can see in her face this is yet another 'mad' thing—proof that I'm not in my right mind.

'But you need the blood test,' she says.
'No one told me about a bloody blood test. Why do you keep springing these things on me?'

She purses her lips and looks at the clock.

'What do I need a blood test for anyway?'

'To measure the sodium valproate levels to make sure the dose is correct.'

I take a deep breath and try to calm down.

'I'll be back by eleven, would that work?' I say trying to be reasonable.

'Well it is more convenient—'

'Not for me, it's not.'

'Come on, Jen,' says The Norwegian. 'We'll do the blood test later. You just have to fit it in,' he says. He takes my hand and we sweep down the corridor.

'Thanks, babes,

I'm really getting to the end of my tether with this place.'

'Me too.'

We walk in companionable silence holding hands, and The Norwegian pushes the buggy. In the large glass foyer of the swimming pool a woman in her mid fifties is waiting at the reception desk. She has short dark hair and a swimmer's broad shoulders. She smiles at me.

'I've come for my lesson,' I say.

'That's me. Come downstairs and we'll get going.'

I strip of my clothes by the side of the empty pool. The Norwegian sits with The Boy asleep in the buggy. He is reading emails on his phone.

'Do you have anything specific you'd like to focus on?'

'Crawl. I only breathe on one side and I'd like to be able to breathe on both sides. You don't call it crawl though; freestyle, I think.'

'Yes. I've never understood why you Poms call it crawl,' she says.

I jump into the water and as it closes over my head I feel a calm settle over me. I stand up, the water running over my head and shoulders.

'Right, so let's do two lengths to warm up,' she says.

By the end of the lesson I have learnt bilateral breathing and I am out of breath, my heart pumping.

* * *

Physical exercise is recommended to all for improving physical health and is even more beneficial when you have mental health problems. The natural endorphins that kick in when you have finished your run, or yoga session, can counterbalance feelings of sadness or anxiety. Most people feel better when they get regular physical exercise.

My sister has had dramatic weight fluctuations over the years of her illness. Before she was ill she was a slender size 10, but years of heavy medication, boredom and no opportunity to exercise have taken their toll, and she is now more like a size 16 or 18. Paradoxically, her weight can be an indication of how well she is because when she slims down we know she hasn't been taking her meds. Now she is committed to taking her medication she is large, but she doesn't seem to let it bother her. A small price to pay for sanity, some might think.

* * *

We make our way back to the hospital and let the staff know we can do the blood test any time. The Boy wakes up and The Norwegian settles in the rocking chair giving him a cuddle. The Nurse shows in a slim Indian woman. She is carrying a large toolbox-shaped container which she plonks on the bed. She is shy and deferential. I give her a huge smile and ask her how she is. She smiles at me as she snaps open the fasteners and lifts out a needle and blood-collecting tube.

'Very cute,' she says nodding at The Boy.

'Thank you, we think so too.' She gets me to sit down on the edge of the bed and roll up my sleeve. There is the faint smell of chlorine as I haven't had a chance to have a shower since my swim. She coos at The Boy as she finds a vein, then concentrates on my arm as she inserts the needle.

'OK?' she asks.

'Yes, fine.'

By the time she is finished she is chatting away in her melodic accent, telling us about her two sons and what a handful they are. After she leaves I jump in the shower and wash off the chlorine from my skin and hair, and we go to get yet another canteen lunch.

That afternoon a good friend from work comes to visit. We sit in the courtyard and sip coffee (her) and gulp tea (me). I tell her a bit of what has been happening.

'It has been really frightening but I feel so much better now.'

'Psychosis, psyshmosis,' she says. 'You seem fine to me.' And I am fine at that moment.

One of the hardest things for The Norwegian was that, for long stretches, I would be fine, but then with no warning I would suddenly become really argumentative. Most days he would go to the park and sit and cry. It breaks my heart to think of him there, alone and sad, because I had raged and ranted about something I wouldn't even remember the next day.

* * *

When my sister was first in hospital in Homerton, I tried to visit her often, though not as often as I should have. I would roll up my trousers and tuck them into my socks, clip on my bicycle helmet, carry the bike up the stairs from the basement of 106 Osbaldeston and peddle to the hospital, via Hackney Downs and Chatsworth road.

I remember the feeling of dread. Partly dreading seeing my beautiful, fun-loving sister so frightened and confused, and partly fear of the other patients. I remember on one visit we were sat in the TV room with one of her new friends from the ward. The room was square with high ceilings. The curtains were drawn and it was gloomy and dark. The TV was bolted at the top of one wall in a corner. There were two young men watching the TV, and one man sitting at one of the other tables slowly flicking through a pack of playing cards. There was a soft snapping sound as he turned over each card and the burbling of the TV in the background.

'Marcel is a good friend,' she said. 'One of the few good people here.'

He had a shaved head and light brown skin. His scalp was rippled and folded as if his skull had melted into his brain. He looked at me with his dull brown eyes and smiled. I didn't know where to look and couldn't meet his dead stare. I wanted to bundle my sister up and take her away from that place, and from that man. I wanted to make her safe. But most of all I wanted her not to have been ill.

Chapter Twenty

Once the long weekend is over we start seeing The Registrar Psychiatrist. He is tall and slim with curly black hair and a youthful face sprinkled with freckles. The days pass with meals in the canteen, walks in the park and sessions with The Psychiatrist. We come to realise that the best place for me to get better is at home among my familiar things, and not being scrutinised, all hours of the day, by the various staff members.

As the anti-psychotic medication starts to kick in, the mania and delusions fade. The Norwegian and I slowly start to get back to our normal, wonderful relationship, defined by kindness, care and understanding—not snap judgements, harsh words and arguing. It is a huge relief for both us, as the days tick by, that my periods of extreme irritation become few and far between, though we get steadily more and more irritated by the staff.

We try to express our dissatisfaction, and they do try and listen, but I have the very strong feeling they are dismissing my difficulties as part of my illness, rather than anything that they are doing wrong. They find it harder to brush off The Norwegian; he starts having to advocate for me, and to be very assertive. They have no choice but to listen to us.

* * *

Over the years my sister has had many run-ins with the staff who have been looking after her. There was one horrible incident when she was being driven to her flat by one of the psychiatric nurses while on escorted leave. She was taken by the conviction that this nurse was going to harm her and, at a set of traffic lights, she burst open the door, climbed onto the bonnet and started trying to rip of the windscreen wipers. She wasn't given leave for a little while after that.

In another secure ward, one of the highest security ones she has ever stayed in, they wouldn't even let her have a cup of tea, with someone else in the room, in case she threw it. One day she managed to smuggle in rocks from the patch of garden they were allowed in, and threw them at the glass of the central nurses' station, with all the staff standing open-mouthed as she raged at them. Luckily the glass was toughened and no one was hurt. Now I understand her frustration and anger as I am subject to the power and control the staff have over me, even as a voluntary patient. I sometimes felt like throwing a few stones myself and ripping that Handover In Progress sign into little pieces.

It fills me with sadness that, whether she was right or wrong in her feelings towards the staff, she didn't have anyone with her every moment to advocate for her, as I do with The Norwegian. My parents have tried but, because of Jo's paranoia, this hasn't always been easy. The most awful thing is that, even if the things she thought the staff were doing to her were one of her delusions, she would have experienced them as real. And the feeling that no one believed her must have been awful to bear in the midst of her muddled and paranoid thinking.

* * *

On Thursday we are walking in the park. The sun is warm and the Noisy Miner birds are calling to each other from the large trees dotted throughout the park. I'm pushing the buggy and The Norwegian is holding my hand. The Boy is burbling away, waving his hands and feet in the air.

'I think the worst is over,' I say.

'Me, too,' he says giving me a tight hug.

'I'm feeling much more myself.'

'I can tell.'

And the worst was over. For the time being, anyway.

We sit on a bench and, still holding hands, we chat about the hospital and the other patients. The afternoon passes in a glow of peace and contentment. That night I'm still feeling so happy and content. We settle The Boy, have dinner and tuck ourselves into the double bed.

'Even though this place is getting to us, we are so lucky really that you got a place,' says The Norwegian. 'Imagine if you'd had to go into hospital without me or The Boy.'

'Don't. Even though we're getting sick of the staff, it isn't as bad as I feared. Nothing like any of the hospitals Jo's been in. But as everyone keeps telling me, I am different to my sister.'

He rolls over and we hug pressing our bodies tightly together. We have a warm soft kiss. One thing was just about to lead to another when the door creaks open and an upside down L of light streams into the room around the door. A figure is outlined against the bright light of the corridor. She is carrying a torch.

The Norwegian jumps up and we both clamp the duvet over our nakedness.
'Who's that?' I ask sharply.
'Just me, The Nurse?'
'What are you doing? It is eleven o'clock!'
'Obs.'
'What the hell is that?' I say.
'Jen,' says The Norwegian. I can hear the tension in his voice.
'Well, we need to keep an eye on you,' she says and closes the door.
'For fuck's sake,' I say. 'She didn't even knock.'
'What timing,' I say. 'Thank God we weren't, you know, at it!'
We burst out laughing.
'Well we are going to have to sleep with PJs on now. No more Mr Naked guy,' says The Norwegian.

Chapter Twenty One

The next morning we ask one of the nurses what 'obs' are.

'You're just coming out of psychosis, so we need to monitor you.'

'Even when we are asleep?'

'You might not be asleep, that's the point.'

'How often do you check?'

'Every hour.'

'WHAT! Why didn't anyone tell us?'

'They didn't?'

'No. And last night someone walked in on us almost having sex.'

One of the other patients is walking past just as I say this. She is a tall woman with long dark hair parted in the middle. She has a long skirt and bare feet. She stops, leaning against the wall just outside the staff room.

'Oh, dear,' says she looking concerned. I wonder if wanting to have sex in the middle of a crisis is another 'symptom' of my psychosis, just like the vomiting and involuntary body movements. It's almost as if anything that happens to me will be attributed to the psychosis.

'It would have been nice if someone had told us. Warned us. It is yet another thing that we haven't been told about. Just because I'm a patient here and not well, doesn't mean we're not entitled to our privacy.'

'Come on, Jen, let's get breakfast,' says The Norwegian taking my hand and leading me away. We walk past the tall woman.

'I hear what you are saying,' she whispers to me with a smile.

At breakfast we talk plans.

'I want to go.'

'I agree. The best place for you is at home. It's doing you no good being scrutinised all day long.'

'We have a meeting with The Psychiatrist this morning, don't we? We can tell him then.'

'We want to leave,' I say to The Psychiatrist later that morning. We are sitting in his little rectangular office. The Norwegian nods.

'Can you tell me why?'

'We think the best place for me to be is at home. We are getting quite annoyed at the way the staff are treating us, well … me, really.'

'Why?'

'Well, lots of things. I have to keep reminding them to give me meds. The handover sign is always up and the door closed, or it seems that way to us. If someone had just taken the time to explain how things work, to start with, it wouldn't have been so bad. But we seem to find things out by accident. There is Group that no one told us about. And, the fact that I'm not allowed out on my own, which doesn't make sense when I'm a voluntary patient. And obs. Someone actually walked in on us nearly having sex last night.'

He laughs nervously.

'Have you been warned about the side effect of mood stabilisers?'

'No, I don't think so.'

'It can cause severe birth defects if you take it while pregnant so you need to make sure you are taking precautions.'

'Surely someone should have told us that, and about any other side effects. I'm not planning to get pregnant any time soon, or ever again, for that matter, but what if we were considering it? That's another really good example of what we're finding difficult here. It's almost like everyone is assuming someone else has filled us in.'

'I see.'

'Also I have the feeling I'm being treated as a collection of symptoms not a person. It seems like everything that happens, or that I do, is put down to my psychosis.'

'Like what?'

'I was throwing up on my first night and The Nurse said it was linked to my psychosis, and then we found out that a few other people had been sick so it was probably a bug or food poisoning. It's like they just discount anything I say because I'm ill. It is a horrible belittling feeling of being ignored, being dismissed.'

'I see,' he says again.

'But the worst thing is the feeling of being scrutinised the whole time. Like right now, I'm talking to you but I know you are observing me and looking for signs of the state of my mental health. It sounds a bit paranoid, I know, but you're not mad if everyone *is* actually looking at you the whole time.'

He laughs. 'Yes I can see how that would be quite off-putting.'

'It is more than off-putting, it is very, very difficult to deal with when I am feeling so vulnerable.'

He nods.

'Though I'm feeling so much better,' I quickly add.' I just want to go home and start learning how to be a mum again.'

'I'm sorry you've been having this not-great experience. We really would recommend you stay. But you're right, you *are* a voluntary patient so you're free to leave. If you can wait till this afternoon I'd like you to meet The Professor who is in charge around here.'

'Another meeting with people staring at me.'

'Well, we'll try not to stare.' He tries a weak smile on me.

I look at The Norwegian and he nods.

'OK, we'll wait until then, but we're really determined to go.'

We go back to the room and start packing up. The meeting with The Professor is scheduled for two o'clock. At five to two we file back into the little office. The Boy starts to cry and The Norwegian picks him up and comforts him. We are introduced to The Professor and a third member of staff who is in charge of the nurses. She has been on holiday, she explains.

'But I'm back now and want to make sure we improve things for you.'

The Professor is a tall slim woman with a prominent nose and brown wavy hair. She is wearing a trouser suit in a soft grey material. She has a necklace of large green beads resting on her shirt.

'I hear that you have been having difficulties and want to leave,' says The Professor. 'This is why we asked a member of the nursing staff to sit in on this meeting so she can hear some of the problems you've been having and see if there is anything we can do to make things better.'

'We are really keen to go,' I say to her and repeat what we said earlier to The Psychiatrist.

She listens carefully with a grave face. As I talk I feel the eyes of everyone in the room boring into me. I rub my face with one hand.

'I understand that you need to keep an eye on us patients, but it's the scrutiny that is just getting too much to bear. The Psychiatrist says you'd prefer for me to stay but I can leave if I want. So we are going to leave.'

'I understand, but I must just say again that we think it is too soon for you to leave.'

'But I'm feeling much better.' How many times had I heard Jo say this when she was still seriously ill and desperate to get out of hospital. I feel a sob welling up. I try and clamp it down. It is vital that I don't cry in front of The Professor.

'You have only just come out of psychosis. You are still in the middle of your mixed episode.'

'What's that? I thought I had postpartum psychosis?'

'It is more accurate to say mixed episode as you've also experienced mania and grandiose thinking, as well as delusions and hallucinations.'

'I haven't had any delusions since the first day, or any involuntary body movements. I think I'm almost back to normal.' I smile at all three of them. Their eyes continue to bore into me. I feel trapped by their collective gaze like an insect in amber. I feel the sob again fighting to get out of my chest. I believed this to be true at the time. I thought that my monk delusion was the last one, but now I realise I was still far from well, even seeing the lizard bird in the courtyard was a delusion. I was definitely still somewhat manic, still occasionally arguing with The Norwegian and having strange thoughts. It amazes me that we did leave that day and managed to cope for a few weeks. That was before the next thing to go wrong, went wrong.

* * *

Over the years Jo has had many delusions. Many were paranoid, like when she thought Mum was a vampire wanting to hurt her, and some were dangerous, like when she thought she could fly and tried to jump out of a window; all were confusing. I was visiting her a few years back when she was in a high-security unit (the one where she threw the stones). She was really very unwell, one of the worst periods she'd had. We sat in the visitors' room facing each other on institutional armchairs next to the institutional pine coffee table.

She was jumpy and distracted.

'How you doing, Jo?' I asked.

'OK, but—' she stopped, staring out through the window. A look of alarm bloomed on her face. All of a sudden with a sharp intake of breath she jumped to her feet.

'The princes. They are in danger.'

'Which princes?'

'William and Harry. They are in terrible danger.'

'No, Jo, I don't think so. I think they have lots of bodyguards.' I got up and held out my hand. She took it and I gave her hand a squeeze.

'Come and sit back down, Jo. Everything is OK.'

She moved back to her chair and we both sat down. She was looking nervously around the room.

'Are you sure?'

'Yes. So tell me about the art you've been doing.'

She smiled at me and the delusion was forgotten.

One of the things I have learnt from my experience is that, it doesn't matter how wild or crazy, when you are having the delusion it feels like reality. It takes a lot of insight into your own illness to realise that you are having a delusion while you are having it. Jo, partly due to the years she has had to bear her illness, does sometimes have this insight and you can talk her down, but only sometimes. The Norwegian has also learnt this over the last few weeks, but still wants me to come home.

* * *

As we drive back home, with the car packed and The Boy safely in his car seat, I realise this is an ending of sorts. I also realise some truths about what had happened to me.

And the truth is: Renée Zellweger isn't living in my building, she hasn't had a child, I'm not Cameron Diaz, Peter isn't a millionaire married to Lindsay Lohan, I'm not going to cure cerebral palsy or schizophrenia, or catch all paedophiles. I don't believe that I travelled back in time to be the first human ever. I have to let go of all these experiences, that felt so real at the time, and I now know they are delusions. All apart from one—that I am going to write a book. You are holding it in your hands right now.

If you, or a loved one, ever find yourself in my position my advice is to remember you do have rights. Unless you've been sectioned under the Mental Health Act, you don't have to stay in hospital if it is really not working for you. You also have a say in what medication you take, and the dose. This is really tricky as the doctors are, most definitely, the experts on medication and it helps if you trust them and the combination of drugs they want you to take.

In general, it is best to take their advice, but remember you are the expert on you, and your personal experience. If something doesn't feel right, then you should attempt to trust your instincts. This is hard to do when your instincts have just been telling you that you are going to meet Barack Obama and catch all paedophiles. But it is still possible. Part of getting better is learning to trust your instincts again, and this is what medical staff should focus on more.

I guess what I mean is that, whatever flavour your crazy is, remember you know *you* the best. Your partner, or parents, or whoever is your support network, are vital to working out the balance between listening to the doctors and listening to what your gut is telling you.

My other piece of advice is, try, if you can, to get yourself a Norwegian. I couldn't have survived the ordeal if I didn't have mine.

* * *

When we open the door to our apartment, and pile the bags up by the door, I feel a huge weight lift from my shoulders. The water outside is a sheet of gunmetal grey with kinks of silver where the wind is ruffling its surface. I sit down in the brown leather IKEA rocking chair and close my eyes.

'Good to be home?' asks The Norwegian.

'Like you wouldn't believe,' I reply. He moves over to me and gently places The Boy in my arms.

'Here, I'll start unpacking.'

I hug The Boy tight and when he starts to wiggle lay out the beautiful knitted blanket, my friend Hilary has made, on the floor and lie The Boy down. I can hear The Norwegian moving around the bedroom methodically emptying the bags and piling clothes into the wash basket.

Now I can just focus on getting back to normal.

'Not yet, not yet,' the Gods of Fate or Chance whisper above me. I still have one more ordeal to face up to and survive. Postnatal depression.

Postnatal Depression

'Where ever I go, there I am.'

My Diary Entry

Chapter Twenty Two

This is the shortest part of the book, though it covers the longest period. Why? Because the depression, when it came crashing over me, squeezing out all joy, all happiness, all light, left behind days upon days, weeks upon weeks of ground-hog-day like repetition. The grinding awfulness of each long, long day was only made worse by the mind numbing boredom, as I found my concentration was shot and I couldn't read; even a magazine was too much for me. But boredom is too weak a word to describe how I felt. It was how I imagined being in a war would feel like: the mix of terror, fear and long periods where nothing much happens, but you still have to be on your guard, never able to relax.

I've been out of hospital for a week and a half when the depression comes. I've been coping quite well with The Norwegian back at work, managing to get out and about, meeting up with women from the mothers' group and my other friends with small children.

On the first day of my depression I go to the local gym where they have crèche facilities. I'd joined the gym a week before and, in hindsight, I probably was still a bit manic. I thought it was all going to be wonderful and I'd get back into shape in no time. You are given an hour and a half of child-minding for less than $6. It is my second time of using the crèche and I go to a body pump class and then have a long relaxed shower after my workout. It feels amazingly luxurious.

By the time I go to pick up The Boy, with just minutes to spare before they shut for the day, he is beside himself, crying and crying. They haven't been able to get him to sleep and once he misses his first sleep, he misses his second, and only sleeps for 30 minutes for his third. He is a crying, complaining baby for the whole of the day, so unlike his usual chilled-baby status.

I'm desperate by the end of the day, totally defeated by the continuous crying. I know some women have babies who cry a lot most days, and my heart goes out to them; I could barely cope with just one day of it.

I push the buggy to meet The Norwegian at the earliest possible moment on his way home from work; he finds a broken woman.

I cry the rest of the evening. Even a Skype with Mum and Dad doesn't make a dent in the awfulness of my feelings.

'How am I going to cope with a baby who cries all the time?' I ask The Norwegian.

'It was just one day, Jen. And you'll cope fine. You're a great mother.'

'I don't feel like one; everything seems just so awful.'

'It was probably just The Boy not being looked after properly by the staff at the crèche.'

'Oh, God, what am I going to do?'

'You'll be fine, babes. I know you will.'

I go to bed exhausted from the heart-wrenching, stomach-churning misery.

The Norwegian is working from home the following day. It is an awful day with me feeling desperately sad and anxious. And that was the start of months of grinding misery so bad that my amazing mum flies out the following week from the UK to help look after me. I am so depressed I can't be left on my own. I am too frightened. My Dad can't fly out with Mum. Problems with his heart mean the long flight is not safe. Also, six weeks is too long a time for Mum *and* Dad to be away from Jo.

* * *

Just after we left hospital I was assigned to a registrar, a Trainee Psychiatrist, and have weekly visits with the lovely Claudette. The Trainee has curly hair around the sides of his head and a thin fringe of dead straight hair brushed forwards over his receding hairline. In our first meeting they told me I would definitely get better. They said all women with postpartum psychosis and postnatal depression do eventually get better, usually by the time their baby is six-months old. Time, they told me, you just need to give it time. We arrange to see The Trainee in three weeks.

But we ask for an emergency appointment after the depression strikes. I know that something is very badly wrong. The Trainee says it is very common to have a period of depression after mania and delusions; the 'up' must be followed by a 'down'. Yin and yang. However, he is very reluctant to put me on antidepressants, despite the severity of my depression, due to the risk of a mood elevator pushing me back into mania. For weeks I'm only on 50 mg of amitriptyline, a very low dose. In fact, this was the dose I was taking to get rid of my tension headaches. I find out later that this is too low a dose to work as an antidepressant.

I still struggle to find the words to describe how awful the period of depression was. If I could, I would instruct the words to fly off the page and lodge themselves in your heart, your gut, and in your throat: lacerating, grinding, slicing, crushing, and stabbing. The words would scoop out your stomach and nestle inside you leaving you hollow, numb and scared. I won't leave them there for long, that would be cruel. I will leave them for just long enough for you to understand how bad depression feels and how much pain I am in.

Days blend into weeks with The Norwegian managing to go into work, despite being heart sick with worry for me, and Mum and me struggling through each hour. She tries to comfort me when the waves of sadness crash through me. I beg to be allowed back into hospital, convinced that's the only way I'm going to be able to cope.

The incredible soul-aching misery makes even simple tasks, like getting out of bed or making dinner, into feats only to be attempted with great courage and support. The pointlessness of having a shower, when you have to have another one the next day, is overwhelming. Choosing clothes to wear is almost impossible, leading me to wear the same collection of things week in week out— a shabby capsule wardrobe for the depressed.

It's hard work looking after a small baby at the best of times, but when you're racked with depression, things can seem impossible. I try my best to play with The Boy, sing him songs and smile at him as I see the other mothers doing with their babies, and The Norwegian or Mum with The Boy, but my smiles are hollow and empty. It is very hard to sing 'If you're happy and you know it, clap your hands' when you are dying inside. I once started singing it to The Boy only to dissolve into tears. I still can't listen to that song without it giving me a chill.

It gets so bad that I finally understand how people are driven to end their own lives. I'd always thought people who attempted, or succeeded in, committing suicide were doing it to hurt others—that it's an act of violence and anger towards the people left behind. But now I've experienced the searing emotional pain of severe depression I have a different view: that for some people the pain is just too much.

All the people around me are saying this will end, hold on and give it time. I don't believe them. The feeling of misery felt so permanent, so forever. Even with this assurance, which not all people with depression have, on my really bad days the pain is so bad I do consider the way out that suicide presents. The thought frightens me so much. But, luckily, it is a fleeting thought, immediately squashed by the horror of the hurt and pain it would cause the people in my life, especially The Norwegian, my parents, my sisters, and most of all The Boy.

Chapter Twenty Three

The most serious of many suicide attempts Jo ever made was 15 or so years ago. I was working in Sainsbury's as a marketing assistant on a temporary contract saving money for a trip to California and Mexico. It was just past 2.00 pm and I was standing at the printer when I heard my phone in my bag. It was Mum.

'Jo's taken a turn for the worse.'
'What happened?'
'Another suicide attempt, I'm afraid.'
I gripped the phone tightly.
'Where is she?'
'In a hospital in Oxford. A&E.'

I had just told my parents I wanted to help support them more with Jo, so we agreed to tag team it, with me going down that day and them coming the following day. I arranged with my boss to take the rest of the day off and rushed to Paddington to get the next train to Oxford.

When I arrived at the hospital, Jo's friends Tom and Tracey were on either side of her bed in a curtained cubicle. Jo was sitting up, propped by two unyielding hospital pillows. Tom looked at me then back at Jo.

'Look, your sister's here.'

Jo's eyes were enormous and her hands flickered and twitched with straight fingers. The rest of her was still and frozen. There were globs of blood on the wall. She was wearing my bottle green VB t-shirt from my backpacking trip to Australia. I was suddenly furious with her. My hands clenched into fists.

How could she? After all these years she is still managing to borrow my clothes without asking. I remember back before she was ill, she had borrowed a favourite top of mine and ruined it with melted plastic from a bag of bread that had got too close to the toaster. She'd just put it back in my wardrobe, melted plastic and all. I remember the almighty row between Jo and Mum and me, with Mum and me saying she couldn't borrow any more clothes from us, and Jo in tears. We'd always been a peaceful family with disagreements sorted out without shouting. That is until Jo hit adolescence.

'It was an accident! I didn't do it on purpose.'

'That's not the point,' said Mum.

'You always leave me out. You don't love me as much as I love you. And you definitely don't love me like you love Jen.'

* * *

Tom took me out of the cubical and we stood in the corridor surrounded by the groans of pain and the brisk nurses and doctors whisking past and disappearing into various cubicles. The smell of hospital—part antiseptic, part fear—crept into my nostrils and smoked up to my brain. Tom was looking at me.

'Did you hear me?'

'Sorry, what?'

'Don't you want to know what happened?'

'Yes, sorry. I'm listening.'

He sighed.

'She said it was just all too much. You know she'd been working in the pub? Well, they found out that she was working of the books and it looks like she is going to have to pay back a ton of money and lose her benefits.'

My chest contracted. He was silent for a moment watching my face.

'She called me. She was in a terrible state and when I got around to her flat I found her passed out, and all these empty medication packs and a half drunk bottle of vodka.'

The anger drained away and I opened the curtain and went to her side. I held one of her flickering, twitching hands.

'It'll be all right,' I said. She gabbled some words at me, looking intently into my eyes.

'What has the doctor said?' I asked.

'None of them will talk to us,' said Tracey.

I pulled open the curtain again and stepped out looking around for a doctor or someone to ask.

'Excuse me,' I tried with one likely looking woman, but she ignored me. I tried with a passing nurse but with no success. After the third attempt to stop someone I began to get angry. I grabbed the next doctor to go past, gripping his elbow. He had short brown hair, thin metal-framed glasses and a square clenched jaw.

'Please, help me. I need to find out what is happening with my sister.'

His eyes darted to my sister's cubical behind me.

'The overdose?'

'My *sister*.'

'I've got other patients, I'll be with you as soon as I can,' and he brushed past me.

My eyes filled with angry tears and I dialled Mum's number on the mobile. If anyone can get the doctor to take me seriously it will be Mum.

'They won't tell me what's going on. She is in a terrible state,' I said.

'Let me see what I can do,' said Mum ringing off.

Ten minutes later the same doctor came to find me.

'I've just spoken to your mother,' I noticed his bloodshot eyes and the pale grey skin around his mouth. His breath smelled of coffee and cigarettes. 'Sorry I brushed you off earlier I thought you were just another one of her druggy friends.'

'What do you mean?'

'Well she has clearly taken some recreational drugs as well as all the medical drugs. Probably ecstasy.'

'My sister doesn't do drugs.' She'd promised me never again after the last time she was in hospital.

There was a silence.

'She needs to be admitted to the psychiatric ward. We're just waiting for the duty psychiatrist,' he said.

'Is she going to be OK? Physically, I mean?'

'Yes, we think so. Her friend found her pretty soon after she'd taken the overdose, from what he said.'

'Thank you for talking to me.'

He rubbed his nose where his glasses rested and closed his eyes for a moment. Then giving me a quick smile he walked away down the corridor.

I went back into the cubical. A look of pure fear flashed across Jo's face as she saw me. I took her hand again.

'Well?' said Tracey.

'The doctors say you are going to be OK,' I said to Jo. 'We are just waiting for the duty psychiatrist. Lucky you got there so quickly,' I said to Tom. 'How did you get in if she was passed out, did you have to bust down the door?'

Tom looked away from me. 'Keys. I've got keys.'

'Oh.' There was a silence as we all looked at Jo. She tried a small smile and burbled something about birds and freedom.

'The doctor also said she was on something.'

Neither of them said anything.

'I'm getting a coffee,' said Tracey. 'Do you want one?'

I stayed for another three hours until the psychiatrist came, and started the process of getting Jo admitted to the psych ward—the start of another of her long stays in hospital. I never find out if she had taken drugs, but being jerked into my sister's troubled and stressful life for a few hours was enough to make me heartbreakingly sad for weeks afterwards.

On the train on the way back to London the realisation of how shit her life was a lot of the time, filled me with grief. I grieved for what could have been, if she'd not become ill, or if what they'd said when she had her first breakdown had been true, that she would get better in a matter of weeks.

As the train speeds along, and with the sound of the wheels on the tracks humming in the background, I rang Mum, crying quietly, 'It was so awful.'

'We should have gone down ourselves, I didn't realise how bad it was going to be.'

'I need to be able to help with these things, though.'

'No, Jen, it was a mistake on our part.'

They went down the next day and got her flat cleared up and her cats looked after by a friend. A sad routine they are painfully familiar with.

I never see the t-shirt again.

My brush with madness has given me insight into how tough things are for my sister. The psychosis I experienced for a few weeks, she has had to live with for months on end. My week in hospital compared to years being locked up for her.

Chapter Twenty Four

A typical day. I wake up, the feeling of dread pinning me to the pillow. I feel completely wiped out from the heavy medication but not able to carry on sleeping.

I can hear The Norwegian giving The Boy his early morning bottle and my mum coming in from next door. She is staying in the spare room of our kindly next-door neighbours as we don't have space in our apartment; our old spare room is now The Boy's.

The soft murmur of voices, as she and The Norwegian chat, filter through the wall. I lie there willing myself to get up and start the day but feel so sad I just want to pull the covers over my head and never, ever get up. Get up. Get up. GET UP. I shout silently to myself. Eventually I force myself out of bed, flapping over the duvet and swinging my feet to the floor.

Then I go and sit on the sofa eating a bowl of Weet-bix. Mum tries to chat with me about plans for the day and I try my very best to answer her questions, and not be consumed by the feeling of misery and dread. Some mornings I have plans, an exercise class at the gym, mum and baby yoga, or mothers' group. Mum looks after The Boy while I get ready. I prepare myself, and the nappy bag, and I'm ready at least an hour before I need to go. I then sit waiting on the sofa for the time to tick away, with The Boy sitting on Mum's lap. I try to fight the feelings of anxiety and waves of sadness.

One of the worst things is, that I feel no joy when I look at The Boy. I love him fiercely but it is a grim, determine, come-what-may type of love, not the joyful, brimming with happiness love that I do eventually start feeling in many months time.

If I have no plans, Mum and I go for a walk, trying to get The Boy to sleep in the buggy. I have sat on most of the benches at Sydney beaches, with my mum holding my hand while I fight back the tears.

We come back to the flat for a lunch of soup and fruit. I can barely sit straight and spoon the soup into my mouth. It slides down my throat and lands in my churned up stomach making me feel sick. After lunch I allow myself an hour to lie in bed. Sometimes I sleep but mostly I lie there willing the time to pass. Then another walk in the afternoon, weather permitting.

The minutes drag. I hear my watch ticking and look again at the time, barely believing that only 15 minutes has passed since I last looked. Each minute is like an hour, each hour like a day, and each day like a week. I wait and wait all day for the sun to go down, so I can go to bed. That is all I have to look forward to.

I'd spent many years doing yoga and trying to meditate with the intention of *living in the now*, being fully present. I'd found, before The Boy was born, that if I was able to live in the now, even for a short time, it was relaxing and fulfilling. It felt like living life intensely and to the full. But what if, as I was finding, the present sucked? Really hard. It left me at a loss to know how to struggle through the days.

It is so, so painful. For me, the depression is by far the worst of my experiences, though for The Norwegian the psychosis and mania were the worst because of the vicious arguments, risk of danger and the unpredictability.

Throughout the day my sadness peaks and overflows. I sob and cry begging someone to do something to help me. My mum holds and comforts me, trying to get me to feel at least a bit better. By the time The Norwegian is back from work we are both exhausted and after dinner I have a few hours where my mood lifts slightly and I watch an hour or so of TV before collapsing into bed, already dreading the following morning.

And the next day, the same things would happen.

And the same, the day after.

And the same, the day after.

And on and on till the days linked up and made weeks. The weeks and weeks turned to months until it was time for us to fly back to England on our planned 'baby tour' at the end of Mum's six weeks. We had planned a three-month stay before The Boy was born, and now realise how much kit you need for a little baby. Of course, we had no idea I would become so unwell.

By the end of Mum's stay I'm still vulnerable, insecure and depressed, but things are at least a little better than when she first arrived. Through grim determination I learn that staying at home doesn't make things any easier. Being out and about, either because of the change of scenery or the company, sometimes helps distract me, and give me respite from the gloom for a short while.

I remember the first break I have in the depression. It lasts 15 minutes. I am out walking with The Boy. There are banks of large structural clouds filling up the blue, blue sky. Swallows swoop and wheel overhead. I close my eyes and feel the warmth of the sun on my face. Something seems to melt inside me. The grip that misery has around my heart loosens. I stop walking. I feel, I can hardly believe it, I feel OK. It is such a contrast to how I've been feeling for weeks that the sensation is totally amazing. I don't know what to do. This is how life used to be. I freeze on the spot. I don't want to move in case the feeling goes away. I stand looking about me willing the feeling to stay. Hope blooms in my chest. Maybe it is ending. Maybe, maybe …

But then, like a cog turning, time moves on and the warm glow fades. The familiar grey suffocating feeling returns. It feels worse than before now I'd had a taste of how things used to be. I turn the buggy around and run back home with tears rolling down my cheeks.

Later that week I talk to Claudette about it. She says that, though it is hard to have such a good feeling come then go, this is what my recovery is probably going to feel like. She tells me I'll have more and more times feeling OK and then they'll start to last for longer and longer. I, of course, don't believe her.

* * *

When we arrive in London, I book in to see my wonderful GP. She refers me immediately to a specialist perinatal mental health unit in Homerton Hospital. They immediately increase the dose of the antidepressant I'm on, saying the amount I was taking won't have made a difference to my depression, as it is below the therapeutic dose. They also quickly wean me off one of the mood stabilisers and tell me it is not recommended in the UK. They say the risk of birth defects is so severe they don't give it to women, even if they're not planning to get pregnant, as accidents can happen. They also refer me to a psychologist who tries to get me to see that I can cope and have been coping. She is kind, patient and understanding.

I make slow, steady progress. Day by day I can feel myself inching towards equilibrium. I carry on my campaign to get out and meet people everyday no matter how bad I feel. It is hard, hard work, but since I have no choice I get my head down and get on with life. I start having hours in the day when the soul-wrenching misery lifts. These hours start becoming more and more common. Some of them link together and I start having whole mornings or afternoons when—I wouldn't say I felt good—but I didn't feel bad.

However, despite this progress, I have regular setbacks and it feels like I'm starting from scratch. I think, *this is forever*, despite what anyone says to me. I have a great reluctance to believe the low period will end. I think this is so deeply ingrained in me because of what happened to Jo.

I see Jo and try to explain what has been happening to me. She is full of sympathy and understanding. She says I am a good mum and a strong woman and will get through this. She comes to stay in London and wants to keep me company. I struggle with this, like I am struggling with everything. I find it stressful to be around her when I am feeling low. I feel I am letting her down in some way.

I want to express to her how I have a much better understanding of her and her illness, but the words come out jumbled or clichéd. I am too wrapped in my own hopelessness to give her any support. She comes to London once and I go and see her twice in Didcot, where she lives. She plans to come down to London again but pulls out at the last minute. We think things are starting to go wrong for her and alert her support team. Mum and Dad are worried, exuding the expectation of impending bad times. Sometimes I wonder about my choice to live so far away from my family. I wonder if there could be an element of escape to it. There must be.

But there are some good times, especially towards the end of my stay. Claudette was right, the breaks come more and more frequently and last longer and longer. I meet up with old friends, get swept along in the 2012 Olympics euphoria, and drink real ale in real pubs. I meet up with my other sister and her family and go to galleries and museums with Mum and Dad. I manage these things still haunted by the ghost of depression. I hang on trying not to get disheartened when the good times turn to bad. I realise how amazing my friends and my parents' friends are. In London I have such an amazing network of support, like a safety net under me, as I walk the tightrope of recovery.

Progress is slow and painful but by the end of the three months I am 80% back to normal, and mostly able to cope on my own. The best thing is that I start to really enjoy being with The Boy rather than being frightened and thinking I can't cope with looking after him.

Chapter Twenty Five

As the three months draws to an end I start looking forward to getting back to Australia and getting back to a routine. I feel we are ready to go back and start moving on with the rest of our lives. But it turns out the rest of our lives isn't quite ready for us. We'd been warned about the jet lag having a potential negative effect on the progress I'd made, so we shouldn't have been blind-sided by the dramatic turn for the worse I take in the first weeks being back in Australia.

The dreaded gloom descends again, obliterating the sparkling sunshine of springtime in Sydney. Checking back in with Claudette and The Trainee I set up a meeting with them for the next Friday morning.

We are sitting waiting outside the office. I am rocking the buggy backwards and forwards trying to get The Boy off for his morning sleep. I grip The Norwegian's hand and tears are gathering in the corners of my eyes. I feel dreadful: numb and in pain at the same time. After The Trainee calls us into his office and asks how I'm doing, the tears start to flow.

'I just feel so awful again. I thought it was over.' The Norwegian pushes the buggy and the sleeping boy into a corner of the room.

'Can you tell me what medication you're on?' He is holding in his hand the long letter written by the psychiatrist in London.

'They took me off the mood stabilisers, said it isn't recommended in the UK, and upped the antidepressant to 100 mg.'

'Well, I think we need to get you back on the sodium valproate to start with.'

'No, I don't want to start taking it again.'

'Is it because you are thinking of getting pregnant? There is no harm in taking it unless you are.'

'No, we're not thinking of getting pregnant, but it just feels like such a step back. And I don't want to be even more tired than I am already.'

'It is about getting you better as fast as possible.'

'I think I just need a higher dose of antidepressant.'

'Yes,' says The Norwegian. 'We think that will do the trick.'

'They told me that the 50 mg I was on was too low a dose to work as an antidepressant. Why did you have me on such a low dose?'

'Let's not worry about that now,' he says then floors me with his next words.

'Bipolar,' he says. 'I think you have a vulnerability to bipolar.'

I start to sob. *No, no, no. I can't have bipolar.* The only other person I knew with that had killed herself the year before. I am devastated. It can't be true. But underneath my shock and desperate hurt I always knew this would happen. All my pessimism about myself, and what my life will be, crystallises into this one point in time. All my fighting, all the reassurance that I wasn't going mad like my sister, all is dealt a death blow by this doctor who's spent no more than five hours in my presence over the months of my illness. Claudette is squirming in her seat.

'It's OK, Jen,' says The Norwegian.

'No! No, it isn't.'

'Jennifer,' says The Trainee

'I can't believe it! This is so awful.'

'You've never mentioned about bipolar before,' says Claudette. 'She only had one episode of mania when she was having the psychosis.'

'Well, either it is bipolar or a major depression.'

'Why not postnatal depression?' I ask, still crying.

'If it continues on past six months then it is no longer called postnatal depression.'

By the end of the meeting we haven't agreed on my medication plan. We insist I don't want to start taking sodium valproate again, and want to increase the antidepressant. The Trainee finally agrees, but says I should double the olanzapine dose (the anti-psychotic and mood stabiliser). This would have put me back to 20 mg, the amount I was on when The Psychologist had to intervene as I was over medicated. I say yes at the time, but thinking about it later that night, I decide not to up the dose. The Trainee says he will get a second opinion from one of the more senior psychiatrists at the centre. At the end of the session he says,

'I do want to apologise about the way I handled this session, Jennifer. I had forgotten how sensitive you are because of your sister.'

I say nothing but just look at him. So it's my fault for being sensitive, is it? I see.

We file out of the room and set up a follow-up meeting on the coming Monday with the receptionist. Claudette comes out of The Trainee's room. She rests her hand on my shoulder and gives me a reassuring smile,

'Remember it is just words. Just a label.'

The following day, on Saturday, I have a session with The Psychologist. I explain what had happened with The Trainee.

'I don't think you have bipolar,' he says.

I feel weak with relief.

'You can see why people and situations get medicalised. There are lots of reasons why you are feeling particularly sad at the moment. I think what's happening to you now is situational rather than biological. When you were first ill, that was definitely caused by brain chemistry, but now I think you are experiencing normal emotions, but just not processing them.

'You have a bad or uncomfortable feeling and you think the worst. It makes you panic. Your challenge is recognising and accepting normal down or anxious feelings that we all have, and not worrying that you are getting depressed again.'

'You're experiencing a lot of loss at the moment. You've lost the close support of your family and friends in London. Anyone would be feeling a bit lost. You've had months of direct support from your mum and when in London from your dad, too, and now you are mostly on your own again.'

'That does make sense. Thank you. But how do I go about processing rather than panicking?'

'You can start by trying to look at the context when you feel sad. Just take a moment, and rather than panicking, think *what is going on that might make me sad or anxious?* Give yourself time to go through options. Then, once you've come up with one or two possible reasons, you can just accept the feelings for what they are. Hopefully this will stop you panicking and help you feel more in control of your emotions. We can work through some of the times when you've felt down and I can help you see the context. It might be hard at first, in fact I'm sure it will be, but the more you practise, the better you'll get at processing.'

'OK.'

'So, can you think of a time you felt sad, down or anxious?'

'Quite often when I'm walking The Boy around I get envious of the childless couples I see sitting on the beach reading books, or just strolling around without a care. I feel so guilty that I'm jealous, almost like I am wishing The Boy didn't exist, which makes me feel terrible, like the worst mother in the world.'

'Right, so we can see that one of your vulnerabilities is a feeling of envy. You must remember it is envy of a situation that you assume to be true rather than you know to be true.'

'What do you mean?'

'You assume the couples you see are happy but they might not be. The couple reading might have run out of things to say to each other, might be bored with each other, or ignoring each other after an argument.'

'Oh, I see.'

'Yes, and the couple strolling might be desperate for children and might, in fact, be looking at *you* with envy.'

'Yes, that's true, they might.'

'OK. Any more?'

'Last week I had a really bad day on Thursday. We had the car in the garage to get the air con fixed. They were supposed to finish on Wednesday but there was a delay and I had to pick it up later on Thursday. That meant I missed two events I had planned: a pool party at one of my friends' from mothers' group in the morning, and then lunch with my boss to talk about coming back to work. It seems like such a little thing, but it threw me into a whirl of misery, and feeling that my life is just so shit.'

'OK, so this example makes me think you have a vulnerability to being disappointed, being let down and possibly letting down others in return.'

'Yes, I see that.'

'So, do you see how you can work through the situation and try and see the context?'

'Yes, I'll give it a try next time I feel sad.'

'Another thing which will help you, is trying to anticipate situations which might make you feel sad or anxious, and trying to prepare yourself for them.'

'OK. So, like, I often get sad on a Saturday morning. I think, because I've been looking forward to the weekend so much, then when it comes and I don't feel as I expect I should, it makes me feel really sad.'

'Yes, so you might prepare yourself for that on Friday evening. Think about how you might be feeling the following day.'

'OK, I'll try.'

I leave the session feeling light. The huge worry of having bipolar is lifted, though it still hovers around me. I also feel like I have more ways to help myself the next time I get sad.

At the meeting with The Trainee on Monday The Norwegian and I stand our ground and, in the end, he agrees to keep the medication at the same dose.

'I consulted with the other psychiatrist who says that, though she can't diagnose without actually meeting you, she agrees with my assessment.'

I sit and look at him. I imagine how he will have presented my situation to her. I find out later from Claudette that she didn't actually say this. People hear what they want to hear.

'Well, that's as may be,' I say. 'But I really don't want to take any more drugs than the ones I'm on already. We think that this set back is due to psychological reasons, and taking more drugs would only do more harm.'

'Well, that is your choice. I just want to get you better as quickly as possible.'

'I'm already taking one mood stabiliser. I don't want to take another one.'

'The Black Dog Institute recommends up to three or four mood stabilisers for treatment-resistant depression.'

A stab of fear slices my stomach. *Treatment-resistant—is that what I have?*

'Nevertheless, we are just going to stick with the increase in antidepressants.'

'OK,' he says.

'And I have to tell you that I didn't increase the dose of olanzapine as you suggested.'

He sighs and scribbles something in my notes. He seems to have accepted that I'm not going to do what he says. I leave feeling more in control.

After we've been back in Sydney for three months I'm feeling much more myself again. I haven't had to increase my meds beyond the increase in the antidepressant. I try to take each day as it comes and hope that soon I'll be totally back to normal. The low days I have now are so much easier than the low days I used to have. In a way, it feels good to only feel a bit bad. Also, the low periods are shorter and I'm more able to take action to make myself feel better, like doing some yoga while The Boy is asleep or arranging to meet a friend for coffee (or tea in my case).

I have continued with regular appointments with The Psychologist. He has supported me in learning how to recognise and accept some of the negative feelings I have, and to anticipate times when I might feel low to avoid getting into a panic. I also have continued to see Claudette. Her calm reassurance boosts my confidence and I look forward to her visits. I don't think I would have got better without the support of The Psychologist and Claudette.

Recovery

'Life just seems so fun and filled with possibilities. It is amazing - I never thought I'd feel like this again.'

Email to a friend.

Chapter Twenty Six

They talk about a period of adjustment when you have a baby. The word adjustment brings to mind slightly moving the rear-view mirror to get a clearer view, or a tiny turn of the shower taps to get exactly the right temperature of water. Not the huge and all-encompassing changes that you go through when you have a baby.

It is hard for me to know what the experience of motherhood would have been like without being ill, but from talking to my friends with kids, they all found the 'adjustment' to be hard, despite loving their children more than anything. These dual feelings of difficulty, and even resentment, mixed with overwhelming love is called ambivalence. Ambivalence is extremely common, but generally not talked about openly. Mothers, and fathers, tend to feel guilty about their mixed feelings. They then hide them from the world at large, talking only of the good times. I had strong feelings of ambivalence, which made me feel incredibly guilty, and added to my depression.

* * *

There is such a taboo around saying how hard, and sometimes awful, being a parent is. It is similar to the taboo around mental health, in a way—not so much in origin but in outcome. This means lots of people suffer in silence. If more parents were brave enough to say how tough it is, then it might not be such a shock when people do have children. More people, also, might be ready to support each other through the tough bits. I'm lucky that I had lots of friends who were very honest about the less-than-rosy side of parenthood. So it wasn't such a shock for me, though I did have more to cope with than most, thanks to my illness. I do wonder how I would have found things if I hadn't been ill. At the time of writing The Boy is almost a year old and my depression is only weeks in the past.

It is quite hard to comprehend before you have kids just how much it changes your life. The sharp joy you feel when your child smiles at you, or rests his head on your shoulder when he is tired, mixed with the unending, monotonous work of looking after a baby—as well as the loss of freedom, especially when they are young—can be confusing and overwhelming.

One of the signs that I was getting better was, even if I was having a tough day with The Boy, one cute heart-melting smile and I would feel full of all-encompassing, bright and beaming love.

The rest of the time just the absence of the chest squeezing and gut wrenching misery makes the days almost joyous. It is such a relief to just feel normal. If you have ever been camping with only cold showers you'll know the wonderful feeling of having a hot shower after days or weeks of roughing it. It is the same hot shower you have every day before work, but it feels so amazing and different.

It was the same feeling for me, something so normal as meeting a friend for coffee or pushing The Boy on a swing, would feel so delicious and wonderful, just because the feeling of dread and misery were no longer pulling away at me.

The thing that my illness has revealed to me is how deep my fear of 'going mad' was, and how much stronger it was in me than in other people with mental ill health in their families. I just thought that the level of fear I had was the normal amount for someone in my position; but for reasons, deeply buried in my past, this fear was huge for me. It is the silver lining of having psychosis, that now I feel that I have experienced a version of madness, and have survived. I didn't have to be sectioned. Though I went to hospital, it was only for a week, not for the months I feared it might be. In a strange way, despite everything, I feel so much stronger and more resilient now.

Or do I? I sometimes do feel super-resilient—if I can survive this I can survive anything. Sometimes. Other times I feel that my confidence in myself is like a vase that has been smashed and the fractures in my being so weakly fixed that the slightest upset will break me again. I have painstakingly glued myself together over weeks and weeks of patient restitution but the result is a self on the brink of falling, literally, to pieces. Each piece of the whole is weakly holding on to its neighbours for dear life. I hope this fragility wears away. I hope that I become stronger than the sum of my parts. I now look forward to my future, rather than dreading the coming day.

Mental illness should be treated by the world at large just like any other illness—no shame, no fear, no guilt—just ill health, which can be treated by medication, in tandem with support from professionals. It is vital any support is a mixture of these two, and people realise, in most cases, there is no magic pill that will make it all go away.

Mental ill health is so common; it's almost a cliché to say so. The Australian Bureau of Statistics carried out a *National Survey of Mental Health and Wellbeing* in 2007 that found an estimated 3.2 million Australians (20% of the population aged between 16 and 85) had a mental disorder in the 12 months prior to the survey. So then, why is the taboo still so strong? To break the taboo people with mental ill health need to speak up and be honest about what is happening to them. That is one of the reasons I have written this book.

Chapter Twenty Seven

The depression takes months to even get to the stage where I can just about cope on my own. Every day is a battle progressing slowly, very slowly. Some days I go back to feeling just as bad again as I ever did, and have to gather my courage and start the process of getting better all over again.

How did I do it? Well I'm still doing it. As I write this I'm not 100% better.

I try to take each day as it comes, good or bad, or somewhere in between. I try not to worry too much about days in the future. I find that makes it easier to cope. It doesn't always work, but I try.

I feel we all need to protect our mental health, as we do our physical health. Luckily, the things you need to do for one, also work for the other. Here is what worked for me.

I have two mantras. I repeat them over and over in my head, especially when I'm walking with The Boy in the buggy. Since I have been ill, sometimes a certain phrase of a song I've just heard will get stuck on a loop in my brain, repeating over and over—driving me to distraction.

When this happens I've found repeating one of my mantras disrupts the annoying lyrics.

My mantras are:

'I am fit and strong and healthy.'

'I can cope with anything in this moment.'

I find the second one to be particularly helpful when I'm feeling really bad. The marvellous Claudette talked to me about 'radical acceptance' and I have found repeating the second mantra is a way to experience this. You try to just calmly and gently accept what is happening to you. Then, because you are not fighting it, or struggling with self pity, it actually makes things feel a bit better. It is quite hard to do, but once you get the hang of it, it works really well. It is all part of something I've been working on for years with yoga and meditation: being present and in the moment.

I exercise. I find this really helps my mood, particularly yoga, swimming and walking. It is hard to find the time to exercise when you have a young baby, but life is much easier to cope with if you can keep active. The endorphins that are released after exercise work as a natural antidepressant.

At the moment I do yoga on a Saturday morning, so The Norwegian can look after The Boy. We do an exercise DVD together most Monday evenings after The Boy has fallen asleep, and before we start making dinner. On Thursdays I do training with two mums from my mothers' group and a personal trainer. The trainer even helps to occupy the babies in their prams while we run around, do squats, sit ups and other exercises. If the weather is nice, and I can fit it in, I also swim once a week.

Most days I walk for at least an hour with The Boy in his buggy; it's good exercise, he gets lots of fresh air and it helps pass the time. Because he is such an active little soul this is the only time out of the house that I can totally relax. Visiting other mums, or having a picnic on a rug, can be quite stressful with The Boy racing around putting bark and leaves, and whatever else he can find into his mouth, or trying to destroy a friend's living room.

I have close times with The Norwegian. This can be a big hug, having a dance around the kitchen or snuggling on the sofa, as well as sex. It really boosts my mood.

I eat well and drink in moderation. As well as exercise I also make sure I eat a healthy balanced diet most of the time. I don't drink much alcohol: it doesn't agree with me as much as it used too. But, that being said, a lovely glass of wine or refreshing gin and tonic on a Friday evening isn't going to harm anyone.

I write. I find that writing every day, if I can, helps. I usually manage to get an hour done a day when The Boy is asleep, though he has started becoming hard to settle. I try and settle him in his cot, but if this doesn't work I sling him in the pushchair, or baby seat in the car, and whizz around until he drops off. This means my hour can't be on the laptop but I bring a notebook to scribble in, or a draft to correct. Sometimes what I am writing is still so raw that it can be upsetting, but mostly it feels good to get the things in my head out and down on paper. It is very cathartic. You might not be a writer but jotting down your thoughts and feelings might help you feel better in the long run.

I get professional help. I am extremely lucky with The Psychologist. He has helped me enormously. He has helped me see that some of the bad or negative feelings and emotions I experience have a context in my life, and are not all down to depression. He supported me when I didn't want to take more medication on my return to Sydney, contradicted my diagnosis of bipolar, and has helped me to see that I have a difficulty in processing emotions, and I tend towards catastrophic thinking.

Earlier this week, after my training session, I went for lunch in a local Forty Beans café. As I sat and munched my way through a tuna mayo and sliced egg sandwich, a family came and sat down next to me at one of the outside tables. There was a woman about my age, with a little baby younger than The Boy, and an older couple I assumed to be her parents. They were having such a lovely time, the grandparents cooing and doting on the little baby and the mother relaxing with a latte.

I am very homesick after our trip to London and seeing this group prompted a huge wave of sadness that I was so far away from my family. Before The Psychologist helped me understand about processing my emotions I would have panicked when I started to feel sad and would have worried my depression was coming back. But, as I know now that I am vulnerable to feeling a sense of loss when I think about my parents, I just sat there with the feeling, acknowledging it until it ebbed away. Recognition and acceptance lead to other options, as The Psychologist has taught me. He told me learning to recognise and accept my emotions is part of a lifelong process, and the more I practice, the easier it will get.

I also see Claudette. It was once a week at the beginning but now it is more like once a month. She has helped me realise no one is happy all the time. It seems like such an obvious thing to say but when she spelled it out to me I realised I had some very unrealistic ideas about myself, and my mood. Some uncomfortable feelings, or sadness, or irritation, is a normal part of life. In fact, we need them, otherwise the good bits wouldn't feel so good. Everything is a balance. Yin and yang again.

I get non-profesional help. It can be so hard to ask for help, but your friends will probably be aching with sadness for you and will really want to help. My group of friends helped so much by just including me in normal activities even though I must have been the worst company.

One of the wonderful things my Mum did for me was write a record of all the good things I did in the day. After dinner we would sit down and she would read them out to me*. When you are depressed you really do see the world through a veil of misery and pessimism. It is hard for you to think

---

* I still have that notebook. It means a lot to me.

about or even remember anything that doesn't provide evidence to back up the overwhelming feeling that everything is shit, that you are shit, that life is shit.

Mum tells me now she was determined to help me see that the real me was still there underneath the layers of depression. She knew it was a monumental struggle for me to take part in normal conversations, but she persevered every day to have light, thoughtful, interesting conversations, like we have always had. If you are reading this and you have a loved one going through PND then try to do this with them. Or help them keep a record of their daily achievements. Both really helped me.

I take my medication. Enough said. Remember you have a say about the mix and dose of medication. You need to be happy with it. Also, medication needs to be taken together with 'talking therapies'. Don't sit back and wait for the medication to kick in. Take an active role in your recovery.

I hang out with other people. Being on my own can make me feel very lonely, so I always try to have plans to meet up with friends and women from my mothers' group every day. Company is distracting but, though it is sometimes difficult just hanging around with such an active son, the benefits of the company of others still outweighs the tiring surveillance operation that takes place anywhere outside of our child-proofed apartment.

I try to remain positive. I've put this last because it is the most important thing to try to do, and also the hardest. I try to believe Claudette when she says all women with postnatal depression get better eventually. I try to believe The Norwegian and my parents when they say they think I will get better. I just need to give it time. This is very hard to do when you are feeling soul crushingly awful, but I really try, and I think it is paying off. Try to believe in yourself and your ability to get back to normal.

And I've survived my biggest all-encompassing fear: that I would go mad like my sister. That I would be locked up for months on end like she has been, and that the fabric of my life would unravel, and it would be all confusion, pain and misery.

I did go mad and I survived it. After that I survived months and months of the grinding misery and anxiety of postnatal depression. Mostly, now, I feel strong mentally and physically. I feel that if, and when, more bad things happen, as is the case with life, I will be in a much better position to cope. I survived and I'm still here to tell the tale.

Postscript

It is April 2013. I finished writing the book three months ago and I've got something to say. Deep breath.

I'm better. 100% better. There I said it.

It feels amazing, but scary, to actually say that out loud. I sit and wait for the Gods of 'Don't Count Your Chickens' to notice my optimism and send me another bolt of depression. But they haven't yet. I think a small part of me will probably always be on the lookout, waiting to see if the depression will return. But mostly I'm just rejoicing in getting my life back.

Life just seems so normal, so easy to cope with, so interesting and fun. I still have times when I feel ratty, stressed and a bit down. But as Claudette and The Psychologist keep telling me this is normal; a totally normal part of life.

Last night I sat with The Boy after he had his milk and I'd finished reading his bedtime story. He is such a wriggler that he doesn't often sit in one place for more than a minute before he wants to be off running around the room or trying to hit me in the eye with the handle of his maraca. But last night he snuggled close and babbled softly to me for – oh about five whole minutes. It was bliss. We sat, me in the chair, him in my lap and gurgled to each other, his face turned up to mine. I basked in the glow of his soft gaze. He started playing the game of touching my lips with his finger. Every time I kissed his finger he would smile and laugh. The most wonderful sound imaginable. I was enveloped with such a strong feeling of love and contentment.

I thought to myself. I've done it. I'm there. I'm better.

Since finishing the book things have been steadily improving. At my last meeting with The Trainee in January he told me I could start scaling back on the olanzapine (the anti-psychotic medication). He said, 'You are officially better – see I told you that would happen.' I looked at him giving me a smug self-satisfied smile. The Norwegian gave my hand a squeeze. 'That's not what I remember,' I almost said. But I was so happy to be coming off the olanzapine that, in the end, I didn't say anything. What would be the point?

The difference was immediate. I could actually wake up in the morning without the enveloping cloud of permanent tiredness. I started losing weight. My intelligence and quick thinking emerged again. I didn't have any return of symptoms, though I did have a few wobbles which were more to do with lack of confidence than anything else. I was guided through by The Norwegian, my parents, friends and the marvellous Claudette and my lifesaver, The Psychologist. And there was one other person who got me through. And that was me.

And last week Claudette told me she was discharging me totally from the Adult Mental Health service and handing me over to my GP who will support me while I decrease the anti-depressants. It really is all over.

Life is so hard at times. If you have a period of mental illness it can completely devastate your life. But my message is not to give up hope.

You are strong, you can cope and you will get better.

Thank you

To my Sydney friends who helped organised day trips to Taronga Zoo, Forty Baskets Beach and Centennial Park to keep me company, and keep me occupied when I could hardly make anything like close to polite conversation: Alex, Vicki, Bhavna and Hannah. You are amazing.

To the women of my mothers' group who included me, and didn't judge me.

To Gema who came around every Friday she was in Sydney to feed me gazpacho and Spanish tortilla before my mum arrived to give me a break.

To Jo R whose 'Glass of Sparkling' therapy on a Friday evening was just what I needed.

To Lautaro—thanks for picking up the cot and for listening to me when I was at my worst.

To Shauna for being totally unfazed when I cried during our yoga lessons.

To almost all the mental health professionals I've met in the last year, both in Sydney and London; you do a very tough job with some of the most vulnerable and troubled people in our society. Thank you so much. A particular thanks to Bibi and Dr Pringle and the team in London; Tara, Daryl and Vicky. My journey would have been *much l*onger and *much* harder without you.

To Lisa who was the first person to notice.

To my neigbours, John and Gabriella who gave my mum a room to sleep in while she was with us for six weeks at the height of my depression, who called the emergency locksmith when I managed to get myself locked out and for all your concern.

To my UK friends who found me changed, but didn't change how I found them: Harriet, Vanessa, Laura, Judith, Aud, Hilary, Emma and Suzanne.

To my new friend Sheya for her kind words and gentle support.

For Joe and Liam for not laughing when I told you both I was going to write a bestseller.

To my advance readers Hannah (again), Bhavna (again), Susannah M and Hilary (again), whose comments and encouragement spurred me on to finish the book—I can't say how much it meant to me. And a special thank you to Hilary for her detailed proofreading.

To Susannah M, The Bunce and Bill for their encouragement, inspiration and wonderful teaching during my MA in Professional Writing at University College Falmouth, particularly Susannah.

To my publisher and editor Caroline, Sonia, Gloria and all the team at Green Olive Press for their eagle-eyed editing and for believing in my story. Any mistakes still lurking in the book are my own.

To Bhavna (again again!) for her beautiful illustrations which grace the cover of this book.

To Gab Maciel for doing the impossible and actually taking a nice picture of me for my author photo.

To The Norwegian's parents for your care and concern, and for generously giving us the whole top floor of your beautiful house in Fredrikstad when we came to visit.

To my parents who raised me to never give up, and who have never doubted me. I feel your unswerving support every day even when we are half the planet away from each other.

To my sister Tania, thank you for the kindness, curry and support.

To my little big sister whose courage and determination have always inspired me. And the parcels and postcards—little reminders of love and care and thought. I love you Jo, Tania, Mum and Dad.

To The Norwegian for always being there, even when there was a shitty place to be. I will never forget how you stood by me, practically and emotionally, through all the bad times.

To my son—the little package of wonder—for his patience when I was ill and love now I'm well.

Support

If you, or someone you know, is struggling with postnatal depression or postpartum psychosis there are organisations which can help through providing information, support or signposting to other relevant services. Remember, though, it is vital that you are also in direct contact with a health professional who can give you personalised support.

If you are feeling desparate call the Emergency Services straight away.

In Australia

PANDA is committed to a community where perinatal depression and anxiety are recognised and the impact on women, men and their families are minimised through acknowledgement, support and education.
1300 726 306
www.panda.org.au

The Black Dog Institute is a world leader in the diagnosis, treatment and prevention of mood disorders such as depression and bipolar disorder.
www.blackdoginstitute.org.au

The Gidget Foundation is a not-for-profit organisation whose mission is to promote awareness of perinatal anxiety and depression amongst women and their families, their healthcare providers and the wider community to ensure that women in need receive timely, appropriate and supportive care.
www.gidgetfoundation.com.au

Lifeline provides access to crisis support, suicide prevention and mental health support services.
13 11 14
www.lifeline.org.au

beyondblue is a national, independent, not-for-profit organisation working to address issues associated with depression, anxiety and related disorders in Australia.
www.beyondblue.org.au

MotherSafe provides a comprehensive counselling service for women and their healthcare providers concerned about exposures during pregnancy and breastfeeding. Such exposures may include: prescription drugs, over-the-counter medications, street drugs, infections, radiation or occupational exposures.
www.mothersafe.org.au

SANE Australia is a national charity helping all Australians affected by mental illness lead a better life – through campaigning, education and research.
www.sane.org

Mental Health Association NSW works towards a society that understands, values and actively supports the best possible mental health and wellbeing for people.
www.mentalhealth.asn.au

Tresillian provides a range of support services to families in the early years, including postnatal depression programs. Whilst Tresillian's Family Care Centres are based in New South Wales, there are similar services in Victoria, Queensland, ACT and Western Australia.
www.tresillian.net

<u>In the UK</u>

Mind believes no one should have to face a mental health problem alone. They'll listen, give you support and advice, and fight your corner. And they'll push for a better deal and respect for everyone experiencing a mental health problem.
www.mind.org.uk

Action Postpartum Psychosis is a network of women across the UK and further afield who have experienced PP. It is a collaborative project run by women who have experienced PP and academic experts from Birmingham and Cardiff Universities.
www.app-network.org

SANE UK works to raise mental health awareness, combat stigma and increase understanding, provide emotional support, practical help and information, and initiate research into causes, treatments and experiences of mental illness.
0845 767 8000
12 pm to 2 am, every day including Christmas Day.
www.sane.org.uk

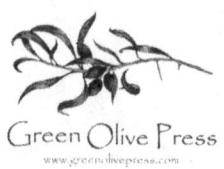

About Green Olive Press

Green Olive Press is a Sydney-based publishing company that publishes 'Stories worth telling, writing worth reading'. Under its traditional (trade) publishing division, Green Olive Press publishes literary and illustrated books, as well as books about food and words. Green Olive Press also provides publishing services to corporate and individuals under its custom publishing division, GOPublishing.

Green Olive Press is the collaborative partners with Forming Circles Pty Ltd for Written Portraits and is a proud sponsor of the anthology.
www.greenolivepress.com